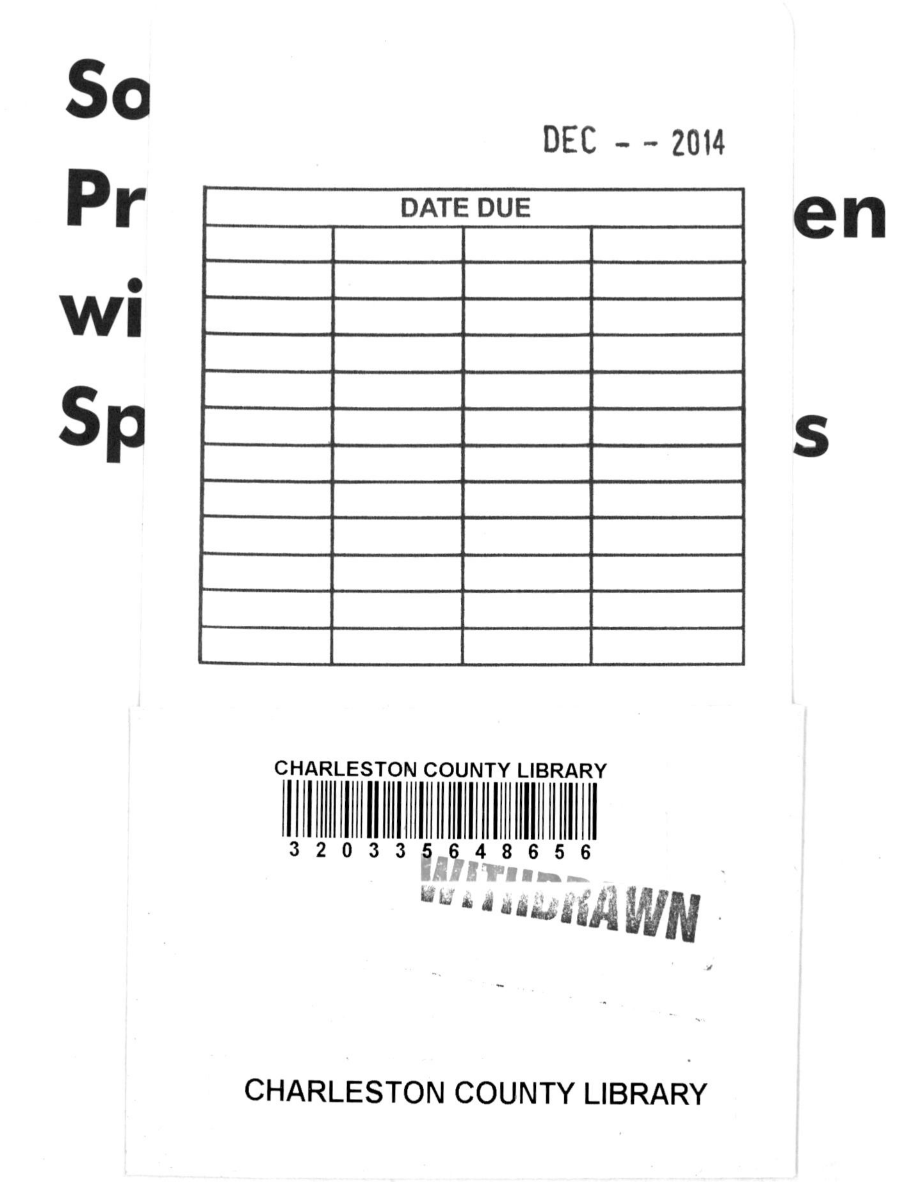
So
Pr
wi
Sp
en
s

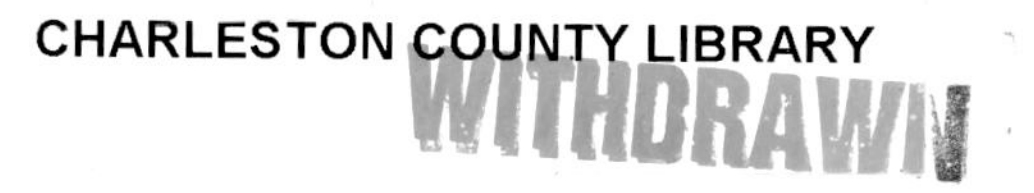

Solving Sleep Problems in Children with Autism Spectrum Disorders

A Guide for Frazzled Families

Terry Katz, Ph.D. & Beth Malow, M.D., M.S.

Woodbine House 2014

First edition

Published in the United States of America by Woodbine House, Inc., 6510 Bells Mill Road, Bethesda, MD 20817. 800-843-7323. www.woodbinehouse.com.

Portions of this book are the product of ongoing activities of the Autism Speaks Autism Treatment Network, a funded program of Autism Speaks, and were supported by cooperative agreement UA3 MC 11054 through the U.S. Department of Health and Human Services, Health Resources and Services Administration, Maternal and Child Health Research Program to the Massachusetts General Hospital.

Library of Congress Cataloging-in-Publication Data

Katz, Terry.
Solving sleep problems in children with autism spectrum disorders : a guide for frazzled families / Terry Katz, PhD & Beth Ann Malow, MD.
pages cm
Includes bibliographical references and index.
ISBN 978-1-60613-195-4
1. Children with autism spectrum disorders. 2. Sleep disorders in children. 3. Children--Sleep. 4. Parents of autistic children. I. Malow, Beth A. II. Title.
RJ506.A9K366 2014
618.92'8498--dc 3

2014008215

Manufactured in the United States of America

10 9 8 7 6 5 4 3 2 1

Table of Contents

Acknowledgments

This book is the result of our extensive research and clinical work with children with autism spectrum disorders and their families. We want to express our gratitude for the opportunity to have worked with these families and appreciation for all that they have taught us. We have been very fortunate to work with families who were willing to be partners with us as we developed effective sleep strategies to help children with autism spectrum disorders sleep better.

A number of the strategies and techniques that we discuss in this book were developed through two research projects. The first was supported by the Organization for Autism Research. The second was funded by the Autism Speaks Autism Treatment Network (AS-ATN), a funded program of Autism Speaks. It is supported by cooperative agreement UA3 MC 11054 through the U.S. Department of Health and Human Services, Health Resources and Services Administration, Maternal and Child Health Research Program to the Massachusetts General Hospital. The Autism Speaks website (www.autismspeaks.org) has many helpful resources for families. A sleep tool kit that includes some of the information we discuss in this book is available on the website, and was developed by our AS-ATN sleep workgroup with the assistance of graphics designer Rebecca Panzer. The Autism Treatment Network/Autism Intervention Research Network on Physical Health (ATN/AIR-P) materials are the products of ongoing activities of the AS-ATN.

Our work with the AS-ATN has allowed us to work with a number of individuals across North America. Much of this collaboration occurred during regular meetings with the sleep workgroup. We are appreciative of everyone's contribution during these meetings and want to thank the following individuals in particular: Drs. Jennifer Accardo, Kelly Byars, Daniel Coury, Daniel Glaze, Suzanne Goldman, Ann Halbower, Kyle Johnson, Ann Reynolds, Margaret Souders, and Shelly Weiss. The AS-ATN leadership was incredibly supportive of our work—these individuals include Drs. Geri Dawson, Nancy Jones, Clara Lajonchere, Donna Murray, and James Perrin.

We are also indebted to the "giants" in the field of behavioral sleep medicine, including Drs. Mark Durand, Amanda Richdale, Judy Owens, Jodi Mindell, and Richard Ferber, whose own work provided inspiration to us for our efforts.

A very special thank you goes to two individuals. Dr. Susan McGrew partnered with Dr. Malow to conduct group parent education sessions at Vanderbilt University, generously sharing her wisdom on how to provide practical advice to families of children with autism spectrum disorders. Kim Frank helped develop many of the materials presented in this book, taught us a great deal about positive and effective teaching techniques, and provided the inspiration to write this book for parents. We are indebted to Kylie Beck for her generosity in allowing us to use the visual support illustrations that she created through her work at the Vanderbilt Kennedy Center's Treatment and Research Institute for Autism Spectrum Disorders (kc.vanderbilt.edu/triad).

We have been very fortunate to have a skilled and caring editor, Susan Stokes. Susan has been incredibly encouraging and has provided wonderful guidance throughout all phases of this project. We appreciated her accommodating our busy schedules and keeping us focused throughout our work together.

We also want to thank our children and husbands for all their love and support. Our children have taught us firsthand about the importance of sleep and the challenges of helping people in our own family sleep better! Our spouses, Jonathan Katz and Stephen Pert, have been unwavering in their encouragement and assistance. We are particularly grateful to Jonathan Katz for taking the time to read this manuscript and provide invaluable editorial assistance. We are very fortunate to have the support of such loving partners during this project and throughout our lives together.

Foreword

It is my very great pleasure to contribute a foreword to this unique and important book on sleep in children and adolescents with autism. Over some thirty years of clinical practice in pediatrics, developmental-behavioral pediatrics, and sleep medicine, I have seen countless numbers of families struggling with sleep problems in their children and, very often as a consequence, in themselves. For many of these families, the challenges of providing care for a child with special needs during the day is made infinitely more difficult without a good night's sleep. And for many of these children, the quality of their nighttime hours makes the difference between a day made more challenging by behavior, attention, and mood problems and one that is productive, successful, and happy.

Many caregivers of children with autism feel isolated and alone when it comes to sleep issues and don't know where to turn for advice and support. *Solving Sleep Problems in Children with Autism Spectrum Disorders* provides that much-needed support and guidance in an understandable, practical, and helpful format.

Based both on the wealth of clinical experience of the expert authors and the existing scientific literature on sleep in children with autism, this book represents the best and most up-to-date advice on identifying and managing a wide variety of the most common sleep problems. By guiding caregivers through the "basics" of sleep in general and the links between sleep and autism specifically, the authors provide the reader with a rich background for understanding how and why sleep problems develop. With an emphasis on healthy sleep habits and behavioral strategies to address difficulties with going to bed and falling and staying asleep, this book gives caregivers the tools they need to manage their child's individual sleep problems, using principles that have a proven track-record. In addition, the concept of a "team approach" to sleep problems in collaboration with the child's healthcare provider ensures that the full range of treatment options is readily available to families.

In my career, I have seen many, many families successfully manage the most difficult and long-standing sleep issues in their children with special needs. While acknowledging the considerable time, effort, and dedication this often takes, the most important message is that your child can also be one of these wonderful success stories. I am personally delighted to be able to offer this great new resource to my patients and families to assist them in that process. This book is your guide to that success, and to making a good night's sleep for your entire family a real and achievable goal.

Sweet Dreams,

Judith Owens, MD
Director of Sleep Medicine
Children's National Medical Center
Washington, DC
Professor of Pediatrics
George Washington School of Medicine and Health Sciences

Introduction

If you are a parent of a child with an autism spectrum disorder who has difficulty sleeping, take comfort in knowing that you are not alone! As you will learn in this book, sleep problems and autism spectrum disorders go hand in hand. We have written this book to provide you with the knowledge you need to help your child sleep better. We will present strategies that have been proven to be successful through research and clinical practice. You will learn about the basics of sleep, why sleep is important, and how to implement a practical and effective sleep program for your child.

There are different ways to use this book. If you choose to read the book from cover to cover, you will start by learning about sleep in general and end by learning how to use specific strategies to help improve your child's sleep. Not everyone will choose to read all parts of this book. We provide an overview of the book below for those parents who want to start by accessing information that is most pertinent to them.

The first part of this book (Chapters 1 to 4) provides information about sleep and children with autism spectrum disorders. Some of you will find this information interesting and helpful. Researchers and clinicians use this information about sleep to develop effective strategies to help children sleep better. You don't need to start with this part of the book if you want to start working on new sleep habits for your child right away. The ideas we describe later in the book can be used by parents regardless of their scientific knowledge of sleep.

Chapter 4 will help you decide what types of sleep problems your child may have and what you can do about these difficulties. At the end of Chapter 4, you will find a list of questions you can answer about your child's sleep. As you answer these questions, you will be directed to different parts of the book that will address your child's sleep problems. Chapter 5 provides information about medical considerations regarding your child's sleep.

Parents who simply want to know how to help their child get to bed without learning more about sleep or even learning about different types of sleep problems can start reading Chapter 6. This chapter explains what to do to help set the stage for an easy transition to bedtime. We have found that when bedtime is easier, everyone in the family is less stressed, and the strategies described in Chapter 6 may help make bedtime better for you and your child. Chapter 7 will give you information that you can use to help your child fall asleep and stay asleep throughout the night.

The last two chapters in this book (Chapters 8 and 9) will help you evaluate the sleep plan that you have developed and apply what you have learned to new situations such as sleepovers and vacations. We have also included an Appendix with a number of materials that you can use to address your child's sleep problems. These materials include checklists, record-keeping forms, and visual supports.

As clinicians and parents, we know firsthand how important good sleep is. We also know that when children are not sleeping well, their parents aren't sleeping well either. We sincerely hope that this book will help everyone in your family get a good night's sleep.

Chapter 1

The Basics of Sleep

Sleep has been defined as a condition that recurs every night, involving both our brains and bodies, in which our eyes are closed, our muscles relaxed, and our awareness of what is going on around us diminished.

You can think of sleep as a basic human drive similar to eating or drinking. If we don't eat or drink, we feel hungry or thirsty. In a similar way, going without sleep makes us sleepy and unable to function at our best. Even though most of us spend at least a quarter to a third of our time asleep (6–8 hours of a 24-hour-day), researchers still disagree about the reasons why we actually sleep.

Why Do We Need Sleep?

Inactivity Theory: One of the earliest reasons given for why we sleep has to do with the advantages of being still and quiet at night when it is dark outside. Animals that are able to stay still and quiet are less apt to be targets for predators or to have accidents. This theory makes sense as a possible explanation for why we lie still and quiet, although one of the problems with the theory is that staying aware (conscious) is safer than being asleep. For example, our early human ancestors who fell asleep may have been more in danger than those who stayed awake.

Energy Theory: In settings where food is limited and needs to be searched for, sleep allows us to reduce our demand for energy, especially when it is harder to search for food (nighttime). Studies supporting this theory have shown that our body temperature and need to take in calories go down during sleep. Of course, this theory applies more to the world that cavemen lived in than to our modern society, where a trip to the fridge is less perilous than hunting or fishing at night!

Restorative Theory: Another reason given for sleep is that it "restores" and repairs what is lost in the body when we are awake. Some of the areas restored include:

- **Immune function**. Our immune system protects us from colds, flu, and other illnesses. When we don't sleep enough, our immune system doesn't function properly, and we can't fight off disease as well. For example, not getting enough sleep has been shown to affect T cells, which play a role in protecting the body from illness. When we are well rested, it is easier to stay healthy.
- **Muscle growth**. During sleep, our bodies release growth hormone, which allows our muscles and bones to grow when we are children and maintains muscle and bone health when adults. If we don't get adequate sleep, growth problems—mainly slowed or stunted growth—can result.
- **Emotions**. When we sleep well, we feel calmer and less "on edge" the next day. In one study, people whose sleep was limited to only four and a half hours a night for one week reported feeling more stressed, angry, sad, and mentally exhausted. When the subjects resumed normal sleep, they reported a dramatic improvement in mood. Studies have also shown that sleep allows us to process and gradually forget events that are hard or painful (or at least allows us not to feel as much pain when thinking about them!).
- **Brain Processing**. While we are asleep, our brains stay active as we think through problems and process what has happened during the day. Using the example of the hard drive of your computer, think about sleep as clearing out all of the excess files you worked with during the day but don't need to store. Sleep allows your brain to store what is needed in your memory, and get rid of what is not needed. Apart from deleting unneeded memories, sleep also allows your brain to clean out waste that builds up during the day. This "clean-up" function may prevent memory problems that can develop with aging.

Related to the Restorative Theory is the idea that sleep is needed for our brains and bodies to develop properly. If we don't restore ourselves at night, we won't be able to grow normally and learn new things. That is one of the reasons why we feel sleep is so important for children with autism spectrum disorders (ASD). They are already working hard to face the challenges of ASD—such as keeping their emotions under control and staying focused on what they are learning in school and therapy sessions. A good night's sleep can go a long way in helping children with ASD perform at their best during the day.

What Are the Phases of Sleep?

Sleep can be thought about as occurring in two different phases. One is called rapid eye movement or REM sleep and the other is everything else—non-rapid eye movement or non-REM sleep. Both are important! There are a few differences between them.

Most of our dreams take place during ***REM sleep*** (although some people remember their dreams more than others). When we are in this phase, our eyes move back and forth as if we are awake. Our heart rate may increase. But our muscle tone drops during REM sleep—this may be nature's way of keeping us from "acting out" our dreams and getting out of

Figure 1—REM Sleep

The top two lines show eye movements, with the arrow indicating a slow rolling eye movement (much slower than the rapid eye movements in REM sleep). The asterisk indicates rapid eye movement. The next lines show chin and EEG (brain wave) activity. Note that this activity is relatively flat.

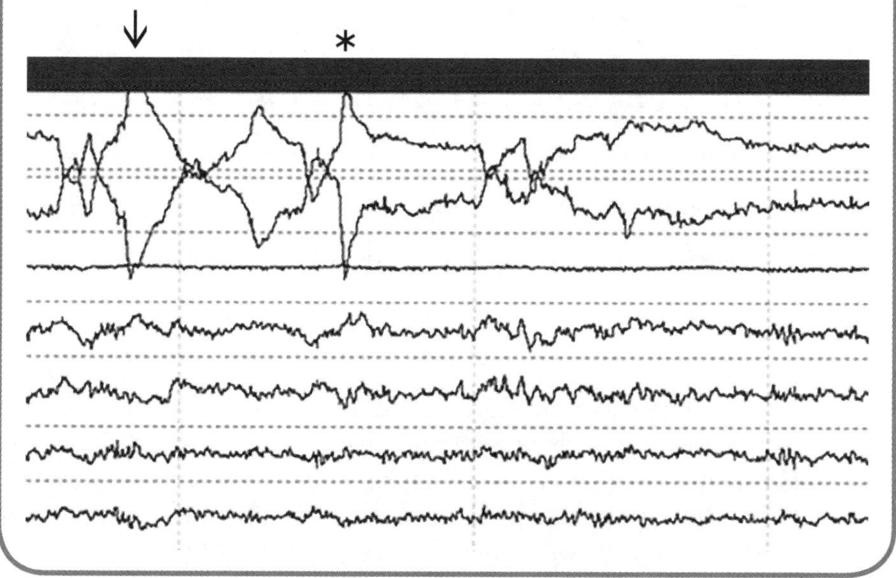

bed and moving around! We can actually record when someone is in REM sleep using sensors placed on the head (to measure brain or EEG activity), around the eyes (to measure eye movements), and on the chin (to measure muscle tone).

Infants start out in REM sleep when they first fall asleep and spend much more time in REM sleep than older children and adults do. Older children and adults wait to go into REM sleep for at least ninety minutes, starting out in non-REM sleep first.

In ***non-REM sleep,*** we may still dream, but our dreams are more like "snapshots" rather than "stories" that go on for a few minutes. There are three parts to non-REM sleep, going from lighter to deeper. The lightest stage of non-REM sleep is called ***"N1" sleep,*** in which we move from waking to sleep and back to waking. During this stage, the eye movements slow down, the EEG slows down from what it looks like when we are awake, and the muscle tone may relax.

The next deepest stage of non-REM sleep is called ***"N2" sleep.*** During this stage, we see two distinct types of patterns in the EEG—sleep spindles

Figure 2—N1 Sleep

The top two lines show eye movements, with the arrow indicating a slow rolling eye movement (much slower than the rapid eye movements in REM sleep). The next lines show chin and EEG (brain wave) activity. Note that this activity is relatively flat.

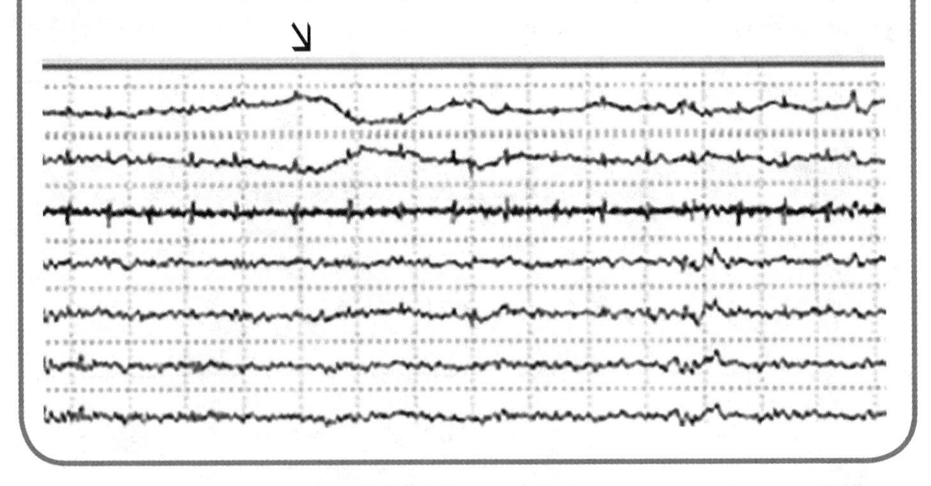

and K complexes. Research has suggested that K complexes occur when the brain senses a stimulus such as a noise. Sleep spindles may indicate times when different brain regions are working together to process information.

The deepest stage of non-REM sleep is called ***"N3" sleep.*** During this stage, we see tall and wide waves in the sleeping person's EEG. Children have

Figure 3—N2 Sleep

The open arrow points to a K complex and the closed arrow to a sleep spindle.

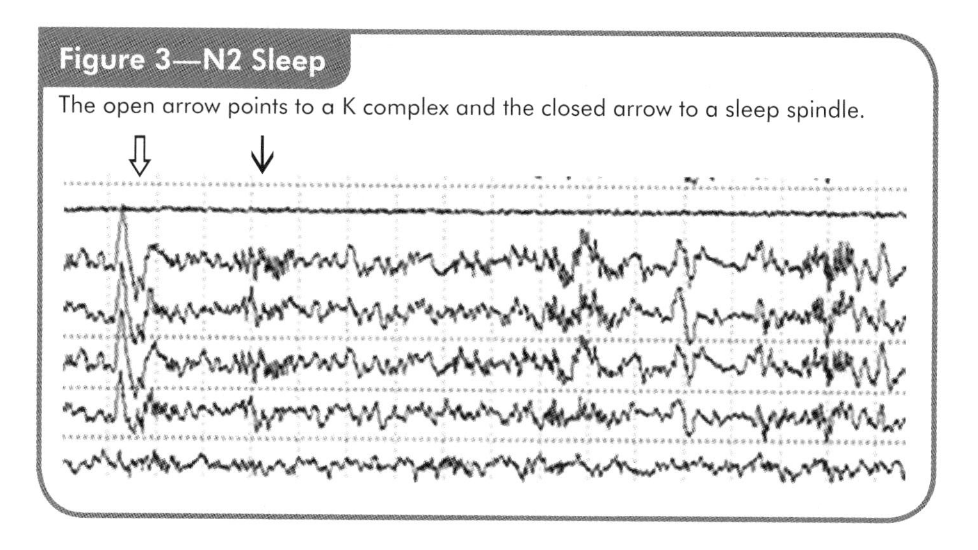

more N3 sleep than adults. This may be related to the fact that hormones (brain substances) that cause the body to grow are more active during N3 sleep.

We cycle through the phases of sleep throughout the night, gradually descending into non-REM sleep. First we enter N1 sleep, then N2 sleep, then

Figure 4—N3 Sleep[1]

The waves are tall and wide. Because of the waves' appearance, N3 sleep is also called "slow wave sleep."

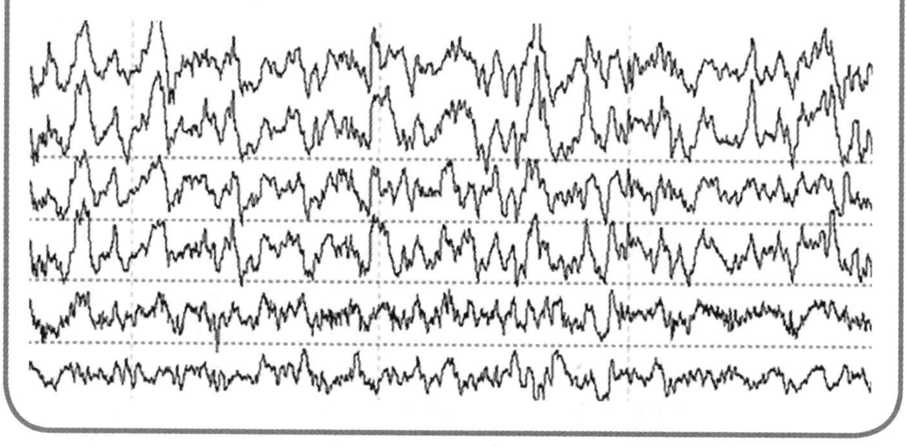

N3 sleep, similar to an escalator descending into a parking garage. About ninety minutes after we fall asleep, we enter REM sleep for a few minutes, then go back into non-REM sleep (N1, followed by N2 and N3), followed by REM sleep. We go through about four to six cycles of non-REM alternating

with REM sleep each night. In each cycle, the length of N3 sleep gets shorter, and the length of REM sleep gets longer.

How Much Sleep Do We Need?

While everyone goes through all of the phases of sleep every night, children's needs for sleep vary depending on their age. In general, children who are in preschool or younger need 11 to 13 hours of sleep a day (including naps), and those who are school-aged need 9 to 11 hours of sleep each day. Teens need 8 ½ to 9 hours of sleep each day. However, everyone's sleep needs are different.

At every age, there are short sleepers, who need less sleep, and long sleepers, who need more sleep. It is possible that children with ASD need less sleep. We have seen parents put a child with ASD to bed very early so that he can try to get the number of hours of sleep that the books recommend. The child then stays awake for hours and finds it even harder to go to sleep! Therefore, we find it better to not insist on a set number of hours of sleep, but instead look at each child's needs. It is often helpful to see how a child is doing during the day to determine his needs for sleep. Is the child waking up easily and not falling asleep during the day while watching television or riding in a car? It so, chances are good that the child is getting enough sleep, even if the amount he is getting is less than what books recommend.

What Controls Our Sleep Patterns?

There are two "drivers" of sleep patterns. One is called the homeostatic drive and one is called the circadian drive. The ***homeostatic drive*** can be thought of as a process causing a substance to build up in our bodies as the day goes on that makes us sleepier. If we take a nap, we use up the substance and are less sleepy. If we drink caffeine, the same thing happens. If we don't get enough sleep at night, we start out the day sleepy with some of the substance already in our bodies.

The reason we don't fall asleep during dinner is that we have another driver of sleep patterns that keeps us awake and gives us a second wind. This is called the ***circadian drive.*** Circadian means "recurring naturally on a twenty-four-hour cycle," and the circadian drive is the body's own clock. This clock lets your body know when it is time to be active and time to rest. When we travel to a different time zone, the reason we feel jet lagged is that our circadian clock is out of sync in the new location—it is light when we expect it to be dark and meals are at different times than our bodies are ready to eat! Our bodies produce melatonin to maintain our circadian drive. We will discuss melatonin further in Chapter 4.

The combination of homeostatic and circadian drives is what helps us stay awake and fall asleep. In Figure 5, you can see a graph with "bumps." The "bumps" are where the circadian drive is causing the person to have a second wind.

For each of us, there is a window of time when we are most prone to falling asleep. This is shown in the graph at about 8 p.m., when the line falls from "alert" to "sleepy." Our brains actually are more alert (and less likely to sleep) in the hour before this "window." This is called the "Forbidden Zone" and is *not* the time to put your child to bed. If you make your child go to bed at this time, he may worry about not falling asleep and become anxious about sleep. The solution is to delay bedtime and move out of this forbidden zone. We will talk more about this in future chapters.

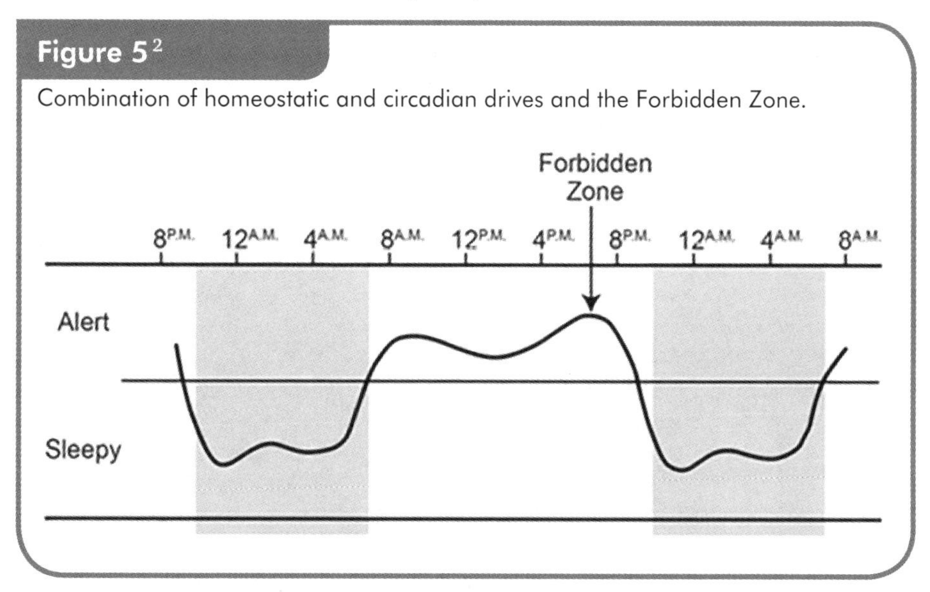

Figure 5[2]

Combination of homeostatic and circadian drives and the Forbidden Zone.

Now that you have an understanding of the basics of sleep, we are ready to talk about ways that the sleep of children with autism can be affected, and how you can make a difference!

References

1. *The AASM Manual for the Scoring of Sleep and Associated Events* (Darien, IL: American Academy of Sleep Medicine, 2012).
2. P. Lavie, "Ultrashort Sleep-Waking Schedule, III. 'Gates' and 'Forbidden Zones' for Sleep," *Electroencephalography and Clinical Neurophysiology* 63, no. 5 (1986): 414-25.

Chapter 2

Autism Spectrum Disorders and Sleep

What is the Connection? What are the Causes?

Sleep is an essential component of a healthy life, just as food and oxygen are. When we don't sleep well, we feel irritable and have difficulty focusing. With this in mind, imagine how a child on the autism spectrum who doesn't sleep well might react. Now think about a well-rested child going about her day at school and participating in after-school therapies.

In this chapter, we will discuss the types of sleep problems that children with autism spectrum disorders (ASD) have, and what the causes are. Identifying the sleep problem and what might be causing it is the first step toward improving sleep in children with ASD.

Research has shown that 50–80 percent of children with ASD have difficulty with some aspect of sleep. These difficulties include:

- trouble falling asleep
- resisting bedtime
- preferring a later bedtime
- waking up at night
- restless sleep
- early morning waking.

Children with ASD may also do unusual activities in their sleep, including wandering around the house or banging their heads repetitively.

It is sometimes helpful to think about sleep problems in children with ASD as having three broad groups of causes, although you will see that these overlap. The first broad group is *biological,* the second *medical,* and the third *behavioral.*

Biological Causes

By *biological* causes, we mean causes of poor sleep that originate in the body. Biological causes of poor sleep in children with ASD include aspects central to having an ASD. For example, the brain chemistry in children with ASD may differ from that of children without ASD. Such brain chemicals include melatonin or serotonin, which play a role in ASD and also in proper sleep. These are difficult to test for, and sometimes we conclude that a child has a biological cause after excluding medical and behavioral causes (see below).

Another example of a biological cause of ASD that affects sleep is insistence on sameness at bedtime. For example, a child whose bed sheets or stuffed animals are not arranged in a certain way may become distressed and resist going to sleep. While it may seem that insistence on sameness relates more to a child's temperament or level of "stubbornness," one of the key features of ASD is a preference for routines over change. That is why we consider this preference for sameness to be biological. The good news, though, is that insistence on sameness can be used to promote sleep. For example, children with ASD are attracted to the use of visual schedules and a consistent bedtime routine.

Just because a child's sleep problem has a biological cause doesn't mean that it needs to be treated with drugs. As mentioned above, using a bedtime routine can promote sleep in the child who insists on sameness. Delaying bedtime until a child acts sleepy can promote sleep in a child whose biological clock is set for a later bedtime. A consistent bedtime can help regulate the natural melatonin levels a child produces, allowing for natural sleep.

Medical Causes

The second group of causes of sleep problems is *medical*. This group includes any medical problem that disrupts sleep. While many of these conditions are not necessarily more frequent in children with ASD, these conditions may be less recognized in children with ASD due to their difficulty communicating pain or discomfort. The list can include:

- ***Gastrointestinal problems*** such as acid reflux. This is a condition in which the stomach contents (food or liquid) leak backwards from the stomach into the esophagus (the tube leading from the mouth to the stomach). This action can irritate the esophagus, causing pain called *heartburn*. Reflux can interfere with falling asleep and cause children to awaken at night. Other symptoms may include burping, spitting up, or vomiting.

- ***Lung problems*** such as cough or asthma.
- ***Upper airway problems*** such as snoring or stoppage of breathing (sleep apnea). Sleep apnea may awaken children from sleep, but sometimes they sleep through the apnea (stoppage of breathing episode). The apnea can still disrupt a child's sleep and cause her to be restless at night and to have trouble with sleepiness or staying focused during the day. Sleep apnea is especially common in children with a dual diagnosis of ASD and Down syndrome, because of their facial structure and the tendency for their airways to collapse. The good news is that sleep apnea is treatable—with either surgery (removal of tonsils and adenoids) or a device called continuous positive airway pressure (CPAP), which uses a steady stream of air given through the nasal passages to keep the airway open. Some children are able to use the CPAP device with little difficulty. Others need help to learn how to wear the device at night. Through a desensitization process, talented health care workers can help your child get used to CPAP and use it with success.
- ***Skin problems*** such as eczema, which can disrupt sleep due to itchiness.
- ***Dental problems*** such as cavities or irritated gums. Dental pain is easily missed and can make it harder for children to sleep well.
- ***Neurological problems*** such as headaches, seizures (abnormal brain discharges seen in epilepsy, which is more common in children with ASD), or restless legs syndrome (leg discomfort that is associated with an urge to move the legs).
- ***Pain*** due to ear infections or other internal pain that the child may not be able to describe.
- ***Psychological problems*** such as anxiety or depression. These conditions can affect a child's ability to fall asleep or stay asleep.
- ...and many other conditions.

The drugs used to treat many of these problems, including antidepressants, can themselves cause sleep problems. It is important to talk with your child's health care provider so that medical causes of sleep problems can be looked for. Treating medical causes may completely improve the sleep problem at best, or at least make the sleep problem better.

Behavioral Causes

The third group of causes is *behavioral*. This term doesn't mean that your child is behaving badly or that you have done something wrong! It simply refers to causes of sleep problems that came about because of a habit that interfered with good sleep. For example, a child who doesn't sleep well during the night might take a long nap in the late afternoon and then be unable to sleep at bedtime. Or instead of taking a nap, the child might drink soda pop with caffeine at dinner to stay awake, and then the caffeine interferes with sleep. Some children enjoy watching TV or playing video games before bedtime and then have trouble sleeping because the TV or video games are over-stimulating.

Many of these habits can be broken, and once broken, the child will sleep better. This book will show you how to identify and break habits that are interfering with your child's sleep.

In summary, thinking about what kind of sleep problem your child has, and what group your child's sleep problem may fall into, is an important first step toward treatment. Remember that you can work on resolving more than one cause at a time. For example, while working with your child's health care provider to figure out if there is a medical cause for sleep problems, you can also be trying some of the behavioral strategies that we discuss in this book.

How Sleep Affects Your Child and Your Family

As mentioned in Chapter 1, sleep is a basic human need that allows us to feel restored during the day. When children with ASD are not sleeping well, it affects many aspects of their lives as well as their families' lives!

Annie is a three-year-old with ASD and night wakings. She wakes up several times each night. Sometimes she comes to her parents' room fully awake and ready to play. Other times, she screams out from her room and wakes up her brothers and sisters, as well as the family dog. She also wanders around the house. When her parents hear Annie's noises, they go to her to make sure she doesn't get hurt and try to return her to bed. Annie cannot get up for preschool in the morning without a struggle, and her speech therapist is concerned that Annie is not able to focus in therapy sessions. The entire family is exhausted.

Annie's story is very common. When a child with ASD doesn't sleep well, the effects go beyond just sleep and may affect the child during the day. Poor sleep can take the form of trouble falling asleep, trouble staying asleep, early morning waking, or restless sleep. All of these difficulties can prevent children from getting the deep, restorative sleep they need to be at their best during the day. In some children, lack of sleep results in:

- problems waking in the morning
- daytime sleepiness or overactivity
- difficulties focusing on school or therapy
- tantrums
- being less engaged with others
- being more cranky and less cooperative with others

Think about how you react when you don't sleep well at night! Many of us struggle through the workday and come home ready to collapse in our beds. Children with ASD who are already struggling with overactivity, attention problems, tantrums, and difficulties engaging with others may be even more affected by lack of sleep.

Now let's talk about Annie's parents. Being a parent of a child with ASD is hard! There are so many things to keep up with, including therapy sessions outside of school, advocating for their children at school, and making sure their needs are met. All of this requires stamina and a good night's sleep! When Annie isn't sleeping well, it makes it harder for her parents to be her advocate because they are tired themselves. As a result of their own lack of sleep, Annie's parents may be more short-tempered and impatient with Annie or her teachers and therapists. Their own lack of sleep may also set up a "vicious cycle" with Annie's sleep problems. They may be less able to think clearly about long-term solutions and more likely to settle for short-term solutions such as letting Annie sleep in their own bed.

The good news is that sleep problems in children with ASD are very treatable. If you are able to put some simple strategies into place, you and your family will see a big improvement in your child's sleep. That is one of the major reasons we wrote this book. As you read on, we hope you will find success in what we share, and achieve your goal of a good night's sleep for everyone in your family.

Chapter 3

Sleep Education

What the Research Shows

This book is about proven ways to help your child with ASD sleep better. We focus on sleep education, which targets children's behaviors related to sleep. The suggested strategies are based on the work of many people who made a big difference in moving this field forward and have provided the groundwork for what will follow in this book. In this chapter, we highlight the major studies that have been done in this field.

In 2006, Dr. Jodi Mindell and her colleagues reviewed the behavioral treatment of infants and young children who had sleep problems.[1] While they focused on children both with and without ASD, their work serves as a good foundation for what we will describe in this book. In their work, they described a variety of treatments that were successful in studies that we will expand upon in this book. Having a variety of treatments to choose from is good, as you may feel that some might work better with your child than others. You may also feel more comfortable with some of the treatment recommendations than with others.

We will provide you with practical ways to put the most effective treatment strategies into place. These methods include:

- **Extinction**. Technically, *extinction* means that you stop rewarding (reinforcing) someone for a behavior you don't want to see until the behavior gradually disappears (becomes *extinct*). In this book, we use the term to describe a method of allowing the child to fall asleep on his own. Think about a family in which the parent repeatedly goes into the child's room to respond to his needs. While making sure your child is safe and comforted is important, sometimes your child learns the negative habit of repeatedly asking for you to come into the room. In "extinction," the parent does not respond to the child's requests to come into his room. Once the child's negative habit of calling for his parent is no longer reinforced, it may extinguish (go away).

There are different types of extinction. At one extreme, the child is immediately expected to fall asleep without the parent present. Using this method, parents never go back into their child's room once they have said goodnight. In other instances, after saying good night, a parent may check in every few minutes to reassure the child, or a parent may stay in the child's bedroom after saying good night, but not talk or interact with him in any way. We talk more about ways to implement these different strategies in Chapter 7.

- **Routines**. This method involves developing a set bedtime routine that includes quiet activities the child enjoys. The idea behind this approach is that it relaxes the child and prepares him for sleep.
- **Delaying Bedtime**. This involves delaying bedtime until children are ready for sleep. The idea is that a later bedtime helps children fall asleep because they are sleepier. It may also be more in line with when the child is naturally ready for sleep.
- **Parent Education Programs**. In studies of methods of treating sleep problems, effective parent education programs taught parents about sleep strategies and described techniques such as creating bedtime routines, developing a consistent sleep schedule, and working with children to help them fall asleep and get back to sleep during night wakings. Many studies also taught parents to put their children to sleep when "drowsy but awake" (letting children finish the process of falling asleep on their own).

In the last decade, research on the behavioral treatment of sleep problems has focused on children with ASD. Some of the key articles are listed at the end of the chapter in case you would like to do further reading. Some of these articles were summaries of research on a few children with ASD, while others included larger samples of children. The common thread that these articles share is that there are many approaches to helping children with ASD sleep. In this book, our goal is to give you choices so that you can choose the strategies you feel will work best for your child.

One of the studies that the authors of this book worked on involved giving parent education to eighty parents of children with ASD ages three to ten years. This study took place at three different centers within North America (Vanderbilt University, the University of Colorado School of Medicine, and the University of Toronto). In the course of this study, we taught parents "the basics" of sleep education. [2]

We found that one hour of one-on-one sleep education or four hours of group sleep education delivered to parents by a trained educator, combined with two brief follow-up phone calls, led to many benefits for children with ASD who had difficulty falling asleep. Not only did sleep education improve sleep for the children, but it also improved daytime functioning including anxiety, attention, repetitive behavior, and overall quality of life. The parents also benefited—they reported feeling more effective as parents and having a higher level of parenting satisfaction after completing the education sessions. The one-on-one and group sessions showed similar levels of success. In contrast, an earlier study in which parents were simply given a pamphlet without guidance on how to use it did not result in the same level of improvement in their children's sleep.

Before entering the study, all children were examined for medical conditions that could cause sleep problems, such as gastrointestinal disorders or seizures. In the instructional sessions, parents learned about daytime and evening habits that promote sleep, including increasing exercise and limiting caffeine during the day. Our sleep educators also helped parents put together visual schedules for their children to help them establish a bedtime routine. The educators discussed ways to help children get back to sleep if they awoke at night and help children fall asleep in their own beds and bedrooms (if the family desired that). Prior to the teaching sessions, parents completed surveys that helped the educators target areas to focus on during the sessions.

As you read on in this book, don't be surprised that what we did in the study sounds similar to what you are reading about! We used what we learned from this study as the basis for our book. Our goal is to help you learn how to teach your child to sleep better—even if you do not have access to a trained educator.

References

1. A. Mindell, B. Kuhn, D. S. Lewin, L. J. Meltzer, and A. Sadeh, "Behavioral Treatment of Bedtime Problems and Night Wakings in Infants and Young Children: An American Academy of Sleep Medicine Review," *SLEEP* 29, no. 10 (2006): 1263-1276.

2. B. A. Malow, K. W. Adkins, A. Reynolds, S. K. Weiss, A. Loh, D. Fawkes, T. Katz, S. E. Goldman, N. Madduri, R. Hundley, and T. Clemons, "Parent-Based Sleep Education for Children with Autism Spectrum Disorders," *Journal of Autism and Developmental Disorders* (June 11, 2013).

Other articles you may find helpful:

Johnson, C. R., Turner, K. S, Foldes, E., Brooks, M. M., Kronk, R., and Wiggs, L. "Behavioral Parent Training to Address Sleep Disturbances in Young Children with Autism Spectrum Disorder: A Pilot Trial." *Sleep Medicine* 14, no. 10 (2013): 995-1004.

Montgomery, P., Stores, G., and Wiggs, L. "The Relative Efficacy of Two Brief Treatments for Sleep Problems in Young Learning Disabled (Mentally Retarded) Children: A Randomised Controlled Trial." *Archives of Disease in Childhood* 89, no. 2 (2004):125–30.

Vriend, J. L., Corkum, P. V., Moon, E. C., and Smith, I. M. "Behavioral Interventions for Sleep Problems in Children with Autism Spectrum Disorders: Current Findings and Future Directions. *Journal of Pediatric Psychology* 36, no. 9 (Oct. 2011): 1017–29.

Weiskop, S., Richdale, A., and Matthews, J. "Behavioural Treatment to Reduce Sleep Problems in Children with Autism or Fragile X Syndrome." *Developmental Medicine and Child Neurology* 47, no. 2. (Feb. 2005): 94–104.

Chapter 4

Pinpointing the Problem

Evaluating Daily Routines and Sleep Habits

Asking the Right Questions

The first step in developing a plan to improve your child's sleep is to answer questions about her sleep patterns. Fortunately, sleep researchers have developed several excellent surveys to guide you. (See Appendix A at the end of this book for a list of these surveys.) These surveys are often used by health care providers and researchers to determine if someone is having sleep difficulties. The questionnaires ask about falling asleep, staying asleep, being sleepy during the day, and sleep habits.

Sleep Surveys

There are many choices of surveys, and you can complete whichever one you prefer. We have chosen to include three different sleep surveys in this book: the *BEARS Sleep Screening Tool,* the *Children's Sleep Habits Questionnaire (CSHQ),* and the *Family Inventory of Sleep Habits (FISH).* Please see Appendices B, C, and D for a copy of each. You may also find copies of each of these surveys on online at www.woodbinehouse.com/SolvingSleepProblems.asp. You can use these to help determine if your child has sleep difficulties that you want to address. At the end of each of these questionnaires, we have provided page references to material in this book that addresses each question.

The *BEARS Questionnaire* (Appendix B) looks at five major sleep areas:

- B—Bedtime problems
- E—Excessive daytime sleepiness
- A—Awakenings during the night
- R—Regularity
- S—Snoring

The *Children's Sleep Habits Questionnaire* (Appendix C) asks about similar areas:

- Bedtime resistance
- Sleep onset delay
- Sleep anxiety
- Nighttime wakings
- Parasomnias
- Sleep disordered breathing
- Daytime sleepiness

The *Family Inventory of Sleep Habits* (Appendix D) asks about behaviors that may influence how your child sleeps at night. The main areas addressed in the FISH include:

- Daytime behaviors
- Evening habits
- Sleep environment
- Bedtime routines

Now let's look at questions commonly asked in sleep surveys. These questions will guide you as you develop a plan to improve your child's sleep.

Identify the problem → Find a solution

What Time Is Bedtime?

This is often a simple question for parents to answer. How parents decide on a bedtime, however, might be quite complicated! All parents are trying to do their best when they set a bedtime. Many parents believe that their child's age should determine bedtime. They think that being a good parent means putting a child to bed at a certain time. They will put younger children to bed earlier than older children. Others plan for all of their children to be in bed at the same time to allow themselves some much-needed "down time." Still other parents do not set limits around bedtime; they allow their children to go to bed whenever they seem sleepy. Some parents will calculate how many hours they want their children to sleep at night. They consider when their children need to wake up for school and put them to bed at a time that will guarantee this much sleep (assuming that their child will actually fall asleep right away!).

There isn't a right or wrong time to put your child to bed! The goal is to find a bedtime that works best for everyone in the family.

When you think about a good bedtime for your child, you want to consider your child's needs as well as your family's needs. In Chapter 6 we'll talk more about finding a good time for your child to go to bed.

Does Bedtime Change from Day to Day?

In addition to finding the "ideal" time for a child to go to bed, it is useful to look at how regular that bedtime is from day to day. Establishing a regular bedtime is a critical aspect of good sleep habits. Many children go to bed at a regular time during the school week, but stay up late on the weekends. When Monday morning rolls around, the later bedtime on weekends makes it harder for the children to wake up for school! It is important to try to maintain a consistent bedtime during the week and the weekends.

What Time Does Your Child Wake Up in the Morning?

It is also best for children to wake up at the same time each day. This is true even if they have gone to bed later than usual. Having the same wakeup time makes it easier to keep a consistent bedtime schedule. Ideally, just like bedtimes, wake times should not change by more than thirty minutes each day. This is also true on the weekends when children don't need to wake up to go to school.

While it is tempting to let children sleep in on days when they are able to do so, "sleeping in" will make it more difficult to maintain a good sleep routine. When children sleep in on the weekend, they will be less tired at the end of the day when it is time to go to sleep. They may then stay up later. If this happens, they will have much more difficulty adjusting to their regular schedule and will struggle to wake up early once this is required. Big shifts in wake time and bedtime on the weekends may make Monday mornings and the reentry back to school much harder.

Getting up at about the same time during the week and the weekend may be hard for parents as well as children. Rather than sleeping in on the weekend, though, we suggest that you and your children get up at the usual time and then take a short nap in the early afternoon if you are overly tired from a busy week. Or, if you crave some time alone on weekend mornings, wake your children and then arrange for them to watch a movie, play computer games, or do some quiet activities that do not require parental involvement.

If it is just too hard to maintain the exact same wake time throughout the week (and it may be especially hard with older children and teens!), try not to let your children sleep in more than one or two hours on the weekend.

Not all children sleep late in the morning. Some children get up much earlier than their parents would like. There are ways to work with children who wake up early as well as those who sleep late. We will address this issue in more detail in Chapter 7.

How Long Does It Take Your Child to Fall Asleep at Bedtime?

This seems like an easy question to answer, but it can be tricky! Many parents are in the habit of answering "curtain calls" or staying with their children for a long time after they say goodnight. This can make it hard to know when bedtime really starts. When should you start timing? When you first say "goodnight" and expect your child to go to sleep. Here is an example:

Melissa puts her son Teddy in his bed at 8:00 p.m. They read together for thirty minutes, then Melissa says "goodnight." After she says "goodnight" at 8:30, Teddy calls out to his mom to ask her many questions. He usually falls asleep at about 9:15 p.m. We would say that Teddy takes 45 minutes to fall asleep.

It can also be hard to know how long teens take to fall asleep at night. Many teens can tell you if they are struggling, but some teens with ASD have difficulty telling you about their sleep. This might be true for a variety of reasons. They may have trouble talking about their experiences and may have even more trouble talking about things that are bothering them. They may also have a different sense of time; while you may think it takes them a long time to fall asleep, they may not have the same perception. In addition, some teens may like being alone in their rooms and may not see this as a problem at all.

Ideally, children will fall asleep about twenty minutes after going to bed. You might want to think about ways to address your child's sleep habits if she is routinely taking more than thirty minutes to fall asleep. Many of the strategies discussed in this book are geared toward making it easier for children with ASD to readily fall asleep at bedtime.

Does Your Child Seem Anxious at Bedtime?

Some children with ASD struggle at bedtime because they just aren't sleepy. They've been active all day, and it can be hard for them to settle down. It's possible that they've also developed some habits that make it hard for them to fall asleep quickly. Other children seem afraid of going to bed. They may be fearful of the dark or frightened to sleep alone. Many children cry or seem uneasy about being in their bedrooms. Try to figure out whether your child is just not ready to go to bed, anxious, or both. Try to notice whether she tends to worry about things during the day or has any difficulty separating from you or being alone for any periods of time. Think about whether she needs a light on at night or wants her bedroom door open and why this might be the case.

How Much Sleep Does Your Child Get?

This is often a key question for parents. They want their children to get a certain number of hours of sleep each night. We have found that the best way to improve the sleep of children with ASD is to work on quality instead of quantity. What do we mean by quality? The goal is for children to go to bed without a struggle, to be able to fall asleep on their own, and to be able to sleep through the night without waking up. They should then be able to wake up in a good mood and do their best throughout the day.

We discussed the sleep needs of children in Chapter 1. If you add up the hours of sleep your child is getting each day, be sure to include the time she spends napping. If your child routinely naps in the car, you should also include that time in your total.

How Does Your Child Wake Up in the Morning?

The way a child wakes up in the morning tells us something about how she sleeps during the night. Try to answer the following questions from the CSHQ (Appendix C and www.woodbinehouse.com/SolvingSleepProblems.asp) about your child's morning behavior:

- Does your child wake up on her own?
- Does she need someone to wake her up?
- How long does it take her to become alert and active?
- Does she seem well-rested?
- Does she seem to be tired?
- Is she in a good mood?
- Is she grumpy or irritable?

Children who have slept well during the night are able to wake up on their own or wake up with little difficulty with the help of an alarm clock or a helpful parent. They may need a few minutes to become alert, but it only takes them a little while to feel ready to start their days.

They are rested and happy. When children routinely have difficulty in the morning, it is a sign that they may be going to bed too late at night or that they may be having some difficulties with sleep throughout the night.

Does Your Child Wake Up Too Early in the Morning?

Some children with ASD wake up very early in the morning and are ready to start their days. These are children who wake up much earlier than their parents would like! This is different from waking in the middle of the night and going back to sleep.

When thinking about your child's early morning awakenings, you want to consider whether this is a new behavior. If it is new, consider whether it is connected to changes in your child's mood or feelings of anxiety. If so, you will want to address the source of the anxiety or mood difficulties. Talk with your child's teacher and other important people in her life to find out what might be causing her to feel stressed.

If awakening too early is a well-established pattern that is not related to daytime stress or a psychiatric difficulty, you can examine your child's overall sleep pattern to determine whether any changes can be made so that she can sleep later each morning.

Does Your Child Seem Sleepy during the Day?

Sleepiness during the day is another sign of poor slumber during the night. For example, it is concerning when children routinely fall asleep while riding in the car or watching television. You might also consider talking with your child's teachers to see if she is nodding off at school. If your child is only rarely sleepy during the day, there is no cause for concern. If it happens more regularly, however, you will want to find the cause for her daytime sleepiness. Children should be alert and awake during the day and should not seem tired or sleepy.

Where Does Your Child Sleep at Night?

There isn't a right or wrong place for your child to sleep during the night. Many brothers and sisters share the same room. Some families prefer co-sleeping arrangements in which parents and children sleep together. There are financial, cultural, and practical issues that affect where a child sleeps, and these are all valid considerations. Children can develop good sleep habits in many different situations. No matter where your child sleeps, however, it is best for her to fall asleep in the same place each night.

Is where your child sleeps a problem? Your answers to the following questions can help you determine this.

- Where does your child sleep at night?
- Is this where you want her to sleep?
- How often does she sleep someplace else?
- When does this happen?
- Does she move from one place to another during the night?

People tend to sleep better when they sleep alone. Even adult partners sleep better when they sleep alone. But this does not mean that your child has to sleep alone. If you are comfortable with your child's sleeping arrangements, you do not need to make any changes. If, however, you would like your child to sleep on her own, see the recommended strategies in Chapter 7.

Some children fall asleep in their own bed and in their own bedroom but need a parent to be with them while they fall asleep. These children may be scared to sleep alone or they may have become used to having someone in their room with them. At times, safety or medical concerns result in parents sharing a room with their children. For instance, some parents of chil-

Children can sleep well in many different places. It is best for them to sleep in the same place each night. They should not be moved once they fall asleep. Children who can fall asleep on their own at the beginning of the night are better able to remain asleep throughout the night.

dren with severe seizure disorders feel the need to remain with their children throughout the night. But even if a child shares a bedroom with others, she should be able to fall asleep on her own. The goal is for her to sleep in the same place all night and not move to a new setting.

How Does Your Child Fall Asleep at Night?

Before you can address your child's sleep problems, you need to understand what she does at the beginning of the night to fall asleep. Think about these questions:

- Is there someone in the room when your child falls asleep?
- Does your child cuddle with another person to fall asleep?
- Does your child listen to music or other sounds to fall asleep?
- Does your child watch television while she falls asleep?
- Does your child need the light on while she falls asleep?
- Does she fall asleep while nursing or drinking from a bottle?
- Does she need to hold a special toy or comfort object?

Why does it matter how your child falls asleep at night? It matters because the way a child falls asleep at bedtime affects how she sleeps all night. Dr. V. Mark Durand coined the phrase "begin at bedtime" (Durand, 2013).[1] This means that whatever your child does when she first falls asleep at the beginning of the night needs to be in place throughout the night so that she can remain asleep. This is true for all of us. As we go through the different phases of sleep during the night, we are more likely to wake up if something has changed since the beginning of the night. If we are able to fall asleep on our own, we can go back to sleep on our own. We can "practice" falling asleep on our own at the beginning of the night. If we can do this at bedtime, we can do it when we have natural arousals during the night.

Here is an example of how this works:

Luke needs to cuddle with his mother at bedtime to fall sleep. This works well for him. He falls asleep quickly without a fuss. His mother leaves as soon as he falls asleep. He wakes up many times during the night, and he won't go back to sleep unless his mother cuddles with him. When he does cuddle with his mother, he falls right back asleep. Luke has learned to fall asleep by cuddling with his mother. He can't get back to sleep unless he is able to cuddle during the night. When he learns to fall asleep on his own at bedtime, he will be able to fall back asleep on his own during the night as well.

Many of us need to do certain things to fall asleep at the beginning of the night. We can stay asleep if we can do these things all night, whenever we briefly waken. Some children learn to fall asleep in a way that doesn't work if they wake up later in the night. For example, if they fall asleep with their parents' help, but their parents don't sleep with them all night long, they can't fall back asleep when they wake up alone. Likewise, it is often difficult to keep the television or radio on throughout the night, so children who fall asleep to radio or TV sounds can't fall back asleep if they awaken in a quiet room.

If we teach children how to fall asleep on their own at the beginning of the night, they will be able to stay asleep all night. Fortunately, it is not hard to teach this skill to children.

Don't feel guilty if you have been cuddling with your child while she falls asleep. You have done what you needed to do so that she could get some sleep. The goal of this book is to give you some tools to teach your child to sleep on her own.

What Happens during the Night?

The CSHQ (Appendix C and www.woodbinehouse.com/SolvingSleep-Problems.asp) addresses many questions about nighttime behaviors:

- How often does your child wake up during the night?
- If she does wake up at night, what time does she wake up?
- How long does she stay up?
- How many nights a week does she wake up?
- What do you do when she wakes up?
- Does she move from one place to another during the night?
- Does she have nightmares?

- Does she talk in her sleep?
- Does she have night terrors?
- Does she sleepwalk?
- Is she a restless sleeper?
- Does she snore?
- Does she gasp for breath?
- Does she grind her teeth?
- Does she wet the bed?

Some of these questions are related to medical causes for poor sleep. We discuss medical concerns in Chapter 2. Be sure to talk with your health care provider and review these questions if your child wakes up routinely during the night. If there are potential medical issues, consider videotaping your child while she is asleep to learn about what happens during the night. It is important to learn whether there are medical reasons for your child's sleep problems.

You can still work on making behavioral changes that might help your child sleep better while you are trying to answer medical questions. For instance, your child might move from one place to another during the night for many reasons. Some of these may be medical, but some might be related to what happens during the night. You can work on medical and behavioral issues at the same time. Your health care provider can determine if there is a medical reason that your child is waking up while you work on making changes to her bedtime routine and sleep setting. She might, for example, be moving to another place during the night because noises are waking her up in the middle of the night. You can work on making things quieter during the night so that she does not wake up so easily. This will help her sleep better even if there is also a medical reason that she is waking up during the night.

No matter why your child is up at night, it is always best to keep interactions with her "brief and boring." This is true even if your child is having a nightmare. It is best to stay calm and be reassuring without spending too much time talking with your child about her bad dream during the night. Save any discussions about the dream for the next day. When dealing with night wakings, your main goal is to make sure that your child is safe and cannot get hurt during the night.

What Happens When Your Child Sleeps Away from Home?

Some children with ASD can sleep well at home, but have difficulty sleeping in a new setting. These difficulties might occur at sleepovers, on vacations, and at camp. Problems with sleeping away from home are often quite upsetting for children and their parents. It makes it hard for families to go on vacation and for children to take part in social events. Chapter 9 covers what to do if your child needs to sleep in a new place.

What Does Your Child Do during the Day That Might Affect Sleep at Night?

What children do during the day really does affect their sleep at night. You want to consider:

- How much exercise does your child get each day?
- How much natural light is she exposed to early in the day?
- How much caffeine is in her foods and drinks?
- Does she take naps?
- How does she use her bedroom?
- Is she stressed during the day?

We briefly discuss the importance of these questions below, and offer detailed guidance on dealing with problems in these areas in Chapter 6.

How Much Exercise Does Your Child Get Each Day?

Physical activity early in the day promotes good sleep. Everyone (not just children with ASD) sleeps better if they exercise at the same time each day. While it isn't always possible to be completely consistent, try to keep your child from engaging in too much activity close to bedtime. A lot of excitement and stimulation right before bed is arousing and interferes with sleep.

How Much Is She Exposed to Natural Light Early in the Day?

You want your child to get as much natural light as possible during the day, but not too close to bedtime. Exposure to light during the day helps keep us alert and keeps our natural melatonin levels down. Melatonin is a hormone that all people produce and is critical in regulating our sleep. It is also called the "hormone of darkness" because we produce melatonin when it is dark.

Exposure to light lowers our melatonin levels. So, we want lots of light during the day when we need to be awake and active and very little light when it is time to go to sleep. Even a brief exposure to bright light can decrease our melatonin levels and make it harder to fall asleep.

How Much Caffeine Is in Your Child's Foods and Drinks?

What children eat during the day may also affect their sleep at night. Caffeine use during the day is one of the most common factors that interferes with sleep. Caffeine is present in many foods, including coffee, soft drinks, tea, chocolate milk, coffee ice cream, some candies, some cookies, and dark chocolate.

The United States government has not produced guidelines for caffeine consumption for children, but there are guidelines available in Canada. The Canadian recommendations state that children ages 4–6 should not have more than 45 mg. of caffeine per day. Children ages 7–9 should not have more than 62.5 mg., and children ages 10–12, no more than 85 mg. For children 13 years and older, the guidelines state that you should multiply a child's weight in pounds by 1.1 to determine the maximum amount of caffeine per day. (Or multiply the weight in kilograms by 2.5.)

Table 4.1 shows the amount of caffeine in some everyday foods. You can use this table to estimate how much caffeine your child is consuming each day. There are many other foods that may contain caffeine, and we encourage you to become a label detective. There are even some potato chips that contain caffeine! Effects from caffeine ordinarily last for three to five hours and can persist up to twelve hours. We recommend limiting all caffeine after 12:00 in the afternoon. Some children are very sensitive to caffeine, and even very small amounts may disrupt their sleep. It is also worth noting that caffeine consumption can also affect daytime behavior. It may make children feel jittery and may interfere with their ability to attend and focus. It might also result in physical problems such as a headache or an upset stomach.

How Does Your Child Use Her Bedroom?

When you consider your child's daytime behavior, also think about what happens in her bedroom. Does your child play in her bed during the day? Is her bedroom used for time-out? For many people, it helps to develop strong connections between the bedroom and sleep. In other words, it is better to keep your bed and bedrooms just for sleeping. If you engage in activities in your bedroom, it is harder to make the link between your bed and sleep.

If your child spends a lot of time playing in her bedroom, it may be much harder for her to realize that she needs to sleep in her bed at bedtime. She is used to playing there and may want to just keep playing.

Using your child's bedroom for time-out during the day can also backfire. Your child may develop bad feelings about her bedroom. She will have

Table 4.1—Caffeine Amounts in Common Food Products

	Serving Size	Caffeine Content (mg)	Check # of servings child has each day
Example: Dr. Pepper	8 oz	28	✓✓✓✓✓ (5)
SODAS			
Coca Cola	8 oz	23	
Diet Coke	8 oz	31	
Pepsi	8 oz	25	
Diet Pepsi	8 oz	24	
Sunkist	8 oz	28	
Dr. Pepper ***(regular and diet)	8 oz	28	
Sprite	8 oz	0	
Mountain Dew	8 oz	36	
CAFFEINE DRINKS			
Jolt	12 oz	70	
Red Bull	11 oz	80	
COFFEE			
Starbucks, tall	12 oz	375	
Starbucks, grande	16 oz	550	
Cappuccino	6 oz	35	
Coffee, decaf	8 oz	5	
TEA			
Iced Tea	8 oz	25	
Snapple iced tea	8 oz	21	
Mistic Teas	8 oz	17	
OTHER			
Chocolate milk	8 oz	5	
Coffee ice cream	8 oz	58	
Dark chocolate	1 oz	20	

more trouble falling asleep if she is upset or afraid. We will discuss ways to keep the bedroom or areas of the bedroom separate for sleep in Chapter 6.

Does She Take Naps?

How long and when a child needs to nap changes as she grows older. Toddlers and preschoolers often need to nap. When older children nap, however, it may be because of poor sleep during the night. Consider your child's age and whether she still needs naps. Eliminating naptime makes it easier for children to fall asleep. Also, consider when your child naps. You should end naps by 4:00 in the afternoon at the latest.

Is She Stressed during the Day?

Children with ASD are especially prone to feelings of anxiety or depression, and this is especially the case as they enter the preteen or teen years. Check to see if things are stressful for your child at school or elsewhere. While it is clear that feeling anxious at night may make it harder to fall asleep at night, working to reduce your child's stress during the day can also improve her sleep.

What Activities Occur in the Evening before Bedtime?

In addition to analyzing daytime activities that could be affecting your child's sleep, it is also important to look at what happens in your household in the hours just before bedtime. In particular, you need to think about:

- What does your child do in the evening?
- What do you do about lowering lights in the house?
- Do you have regular evening routines?

Evening Activities Set the Stage for Bedtime

It is best if children take part in easy *and* relaxing activities about an hour before their bedtime. Your child will be more ready for sleep if she has had a chance to wind down before she starts getting ready for bed. While having your child engage in a lot of physical activity right before bed might seem to make sense, this usually backfires. Too much exercise or activity too close to bedtime can make it hard for children to fall asleep.

Think about whether your child is involved in tasks that are difficult or energizing in the hour before bedtime. If possible, help her become involved in soothing and calming activities. Keep in mind that even if an activity is easy, it may not be a good late-evening activity. For example, watching a scary program is easy but may be too arousing for your child. Think about when your child is involved in stimulating activities. Do these occur too close to bedtime? If you have a teen, you should think about her computer and cell phone use in the evening. While it might not be possible to limit these activities all together, setting aside some time before bed for your child to be "unplugged" may help promote better sleep. Think about adding some calming routines to your child's evening activities such as a soothing massage with lotion, deep breathing, or even some relaxing yoga positions.

What Do You Do about Lights in the House?

Lights in the house should be turned down as low as possible about an hour before bedtime. As we have learned, nighttime exposure to light can really interfere with sleep. Light can come from many different sources. Television sets, computers, and other electronic devices put out a lot of light and should also be limited during the hour before bed.

A recent study[2] showed that using an iPad set at maximum brightness for at least two hours suppresses the normal nighttime release of melatonin. As mentioned above, melatonin production is a critical factor in helping us fall asleep at night. Clearly, it would be best to limit your child's use of iPads (and similar devices) the hour before bedtime, but you can also install products that will dim your computer screen. Some of these programs will even automatically dim your screen based on the time of day.

What Types of Evening Routines Do You Have?

What does your child do each evening? Does she have any regular habits during the evening hours? When does she finish her homework? What about other activities such as bathing, washing hair, and brushing teeth? Many children with autism spectrum disorders have sensory issues. These difficulties often make it harder to complete self-care activities that often occur right before bed. For example, many children with ASD have a difficult time with tooth brushing. If your child becomes upset and aroused during these activities, this can interfere with falling asleep at night. Completing homework can also be hard and may increase stress and alertness. Try to schedule activities that are harder for your child earlier in the evening so that she has a chance to relax once these tasks are finished.

What is your child's bedtime routine?

Here are some questions to consider:

- When does your child's bedtime routine start?
- How long does it last?
- What are the activities in her bedtime routine?
- How many activities are part of her routine?
- Are the activities calm and relaxing?
- Does she complete the same activities each night?
- Does she do each activity in the same order?

We have found that it is beneficial for children to follow a consistent routine each night before bed. We will discuss ways to develop a successful bedtime routine for children with autism spectrum disorders in Chapter 6. It is also important to start bedtime routines at about the same time each night. A good bedtime routine lasts between fifteen and thirty minutes and includes just a few activities that are easy, calm, and relaxing. Children should complete the bedtime routine every night, and complete each activity in the routine in the same order.

How Would You Describe Your Child's Sleep Setting?

You will want to make your child's sleep setting as comfortable as possible. To do so, you want to consider the following factors:

- temperature
- textures
- scents
- sounds
- light
- objects
- people

We discuss each of these elements below. After you have read about these aspects of your child's sleep environment, you might want to think about any changes that might help her sleep better. If you are not sure about how your child might react to these things, try to notice how she responds during the day. If possible, you might also take a few minutes by yourself to lie down in your child's bedroom and think about how she might react to the above factors. You may notice smells or sounds that you may not have considered in the past. Perhaps you will hear the floor creak when other people in the family are walking around in the house. Or you might notice that your child's plastic mattress cover makes a rustling sound when you turn over.

Temperature

Sleep researchers have determined that the temperature of our sleep area affects sleep. Most people seem to sleep better in a room that is cool. You want to make sure that your child is sleeping at a temperature that is comfortable and promotes sleep. It is easier to sleep in a cooler room, but it is also important that the room temperature feels good to your child. It is hard to recommend a specific room temperature, since different people find different temperatures more or less comfortable. In general, a room temperature of between 65 and 72 degrees Fahrenheit is comfortable for many people. You might also think about adjusting the temperature depending on how many blankets your child uses at night. Some children like to sleep with lots of blankets or one heavy blanket. If this is the case, for your child, you might make her room a little cooler so that she isn't too warm.

Textures

Think about your child's pajamas and bedding. While some children like to sleep with lots of layers, others don't. Some children prefer particular fabrics and may dislike clothing that is either too tight or loose fitting. Also consider whether your child is bothered by tags, seams, or waistbands on her pajamas. And think about whether certain patterns on your child's bedding are comforting or energizing. Some children feel good sleeping on sheets that represent some of their special interests while other children get too excited by bedding with special pictures. Knowing about these preferences can help you make your child's bed a comfy and restful place.

Scents

Are there certain aromas that are pleasing for your child? Are there any smells that are distressing? Children with ASD may be much more sensitive to scents than other children, and it may be useful to think about ways to use fragrances to help promote good sleep. Linking a specific scent to bedtime, for example, may be soothing and may give your child another clue that it is time for bed. You might also think about the detergent you use to wash your child's bedding. She may be bothered by the scent and may do better with sheets that are washed with fragrance-free detergent.

Sounds

Most children sleep best in a quiet room. Consider what your child might be hearing when she is trying to fall asleep and what sounds she could be hearing during the night. Children with ASD are often more aware of some sounds than other children, and they may be bothered more by these sounds. If your child is hearing noises from the television, radio, or other sources, it may be harder for her to fall asleep. She might also wake up during the night once these noises stop. Ordinary household noises might also cause some distress.

Your child may be a very light sleeper. Even when all seems quiet, she may wake up to small noises in the night. You'll want to think about what sounds are comforting for your child and what sounds might be interfering with her sleep.

Light

Lights should be off or very low during the night, although using a night-light is fine. Try to keep the lights off even if your child wakes up during the night. Remember to consider lights that are in or near your child's bedroom. These sources may include electronic equipment, street lamps, outdoor lighting, and lights from other rooms in the house.

Objects

What is in your child's bedroom? Are there toys nearby? Is there a television in the room? What about computers? Some children can sleep with these objects in their room. Other children find it too exciting to know that a favorite toy or object is right near them. You might need to remove some objects at bedtime. Some children with autism spectrum disorders need to bring many objects with them to bed. Think about whether this habit is interfering with your child's sleep.

People

Many children sleep with someone else in their bedroom. This is often a brother or sister. Other family members may also need to share a room with your child. Many children, whether or not they have an ASD diagnosis, like having someone sleep in their bedroom. As long as everyone is sleeping well, sharing a bedroom is not a problem. If your child is having trouble sleeping, you may want to think about whether your child's sleeping partner does something that keeps your child up. Are brothers and sisters talking to each other when they are in the room? Is someone listening to music or playing a video game?

You might consider putting your children to bed at different times so that one child is going to bed after another child is already asleep. Putting up a screen between people who share a bedroom might also help. Setting up clear rules and providing rewards for following bedtime routines also works. You might, for example, tell your children "no talking after lights are out" and give them rewards in the morning for following this rule. Chapters 6 and 7 provide more information about children who need to snuggle or cuddle with someone to fall asleep.

Now that we've looked at your child's sleep habits in detail, we can start to make plans to help your child sleep better. We will talk about ways to make changes in the following chapters.

References

1. V. M. Durand, *Sleep Better! A Guide to Improving Sleep for Children with Special Needs*, rev. ed. (Baltimore: Paul H. Brookes, 2013), 111–12.
2. B. Wood, M. S. Rea, B. Plitnick, and M. G. Figueiro, "Light Level and Duration of Exposure Determine the Impact of Self-luminous Tablets on Melatonin Suppression," *Applied Ergonomics* 44, no. 2 (March 2013): 237–40.

Chapter 5

Partnering with Your Child's Health Care Provider

Scott is a six-year-old boy with autism spectrum disorder (ASD). He fell asleep easily at night, but snored loudly and woke up several times a night. His parents put some strategies in place to help him fall back to sleep, but he would wake up an hour later.

His parents talked with Scott's health care provider, who recommended he see a sleep specialist. The sleep specialist talked with Scott's parents and examined Scott. She ordered a sleep study, which showed that Scott had sleep apnea, a condition in which someone periodically stops breathing at night for periods of at least two breaths. Snoring can be a sign of sleep apnea and closing down of the airway. It turned out that Scott had enlarged tonsils that were blocking his airway, and when these were removed, he started sleeping through the night.

Jennifer is a five-year-old girl with ASD. She is scared to go to sleep at night because she is afraid of monsters lurking in her closet. She admits to being fearful during the day as well. She is afraid of being left alone at kindergarten. When she goes for a walk during the day, she is afraid the neighborhood dogs will go through their electric fences and attack her. While her parents have tried to improve Jennifer's sleep by involving her in a calming bedtime routine that involves coloring and reading (two of her favorite activities), she gets more and more scared as bedtime approaches.

Her parents talked with Jennifer's health care provider, who recommended they see a child psychiatrist for anxiety. The psychiatrist prescribed a small dose of medication to treat Jennifer's anxiety. Jennifer also meets with a counselor once a week to address her fears. The therapist is using strategies such as cognitive behavioral therapy to help Jennifer. The cognitive part is helping Jennifer change how she perceives her fears and the behavioral part is working on deep breathing and other strategies to help her become calm. Jennifer is now falling asleep easily and sleeping through the night.

The strategies in this book focus on educational techniques to help your child with ASD sleep better. As mentioned in Chapter 2, however, some causes of poor sleep in children with ASD are medical. If these problems are not addressed, a major "piece of the puzzle" needed to understand why your child isn't sleeping well will be missing! The stories of Scott and Jennifer above are good examples of why it is important to partner with your child's health care provider.

Working with a Medical Professional

We encourage you to talk with your child's health care provider if you have concerns about your child's sleep and even show her this book. Let your provider know that you are actively working to help your child sleep better, and want to work as a team together. Your provider has lots of experience in looking for medical issues that children with ASD may have, with many of these issues affecting sleep. These can include gastrointestinal problems, skin problems, anxiety, sleep disorders (such as sleep apnea), and many other causes (see Chapter 2).

After your child's health care provider talks with you and your child and examines him, the next course of action can be decided. This may include several different paths. Your health care provider may...

- Consult with a medical specialist. This may be a sleep specialist (to look for sleep disorders such as apnea), a gastroenterologist or GI specialist (to look for GI causes of sleep problems), or even a dentist, if tooth pain may be affecting sleep.

- Order a test, such as a sleep study to look for sleep apnea or blood work to look for iron deficiency.
- Start a medication, such as iron or melatonin. There are other medications that can promote sleep as well.

After the tests or visit to a specialist is completed, or a medication is started, your health care provider should meet with you again to discuss next steps. During this time, it is fine to continue to read this book and put different strategies into place. These strategies will not hurt your child. However, after you have addressed any medical issues with your child's health care provider, you may find that the strategies you are learning and putting into place will work better.

It is beyond the scope of this book to delve into every possible medical problem that can interfere with a child's sleep. The sections below, however, cover some of the medical problems that we have personally seen diagnosed in children with ASD who were having difficulties with sleep.

Parasomnias

Peter is a five-year-old boy with ASD. Every few months, he has an episode in which he wakes up screaming about two hours after falling asleep. His parents cannot easily console him, and report that he bolts upright in bed with his eyes open, even though he still seems to be asleep. He does not recall having these episodes. Both of his parents were sleepwalkers as children.

His parents talked with Peter's health care provider, who felt the episodes were most consistent with sleep terrors. Sleep terrors are a form of parasomnia or unusual behavior in sleep. Because the episodes were not frequent, the pediatrician reassured Peter's family that the sleep terrors were benign and he would likely grow out of them. He emphasized the need to make sure Peter was safe when he was having a sleep terror.

Parasomnias are more common in childhood and can run in families. It is not clear if they are more common in children with ASD. Other types of parasomnias that are similar to sleep terrors are sleepwalking (which is exactly that—walking in your sleep!) and confusional arousals (in which a child may wake up in response to a loud noise or an urge to use the bathroom, act confused, and go back to sleep).

Sometimes parasomnias can occur when a child is getting less sleep than usual or there is a lot of activity in the house, such as around holidays.

The most important thing is to be sure the child is safe and is not going to fall or get into things that can harm him. Many parents put bells on the child's door to alert them if their child starts to wander out of the bedroom. Child-proofing the stairs with gates is also important. As children get older, the number of events decreases and usually disappears by the teenage years or adulthood.

Sometimes epileptic seizures can look like parasomnias. If the child does the same thing every time he has an episode, such as stretching out an arm, moving his head or eyes in a certain way, or stiffening and shaking, this may indicate a seizure. In this case, the pediatrician may want to make a referral to an epilepsy specialist for more testing. Children with ASD are more likely than other children to have seizures, but not necessarily to have them at night or to have any specific type of seizure.

Delayed Sleep-Phase Syndrome

Marie is a thirteen-year-old girl with ASD. For the last year, she has had difficulty falling asleep and tends to stay up past midnight. She states that she is not tired earlier. She has trouble waking up for school, which starts at 7:30 a.m. Other family members also preferred later bedtimes, especially in their teen years. Her sleep habits are otherwise good—she doesn't use caffeine, she jogs after school, and she reads a relaxing book in the evening before bed. She does not use the computer within an hour of bedtime.

Marie's health care provider diagnosed her with delayed sleep phase syndrome—her body was just not ready to sleep at bedtime because her biological clock was out of sync. Even with Marie paying attention to her sleep habits, she still had problems. The treatment that worked best for Marie was getting light in the mornings. She switched her jogging time to the mornings to increase her light exposure earlier in the day.

This condition results from our biological clocks (circadian rhythms) being delayed. The person's sleep is otherwise normal—it is just that the start time and end time of sleep (the phase) is delayed. Like the parasomnias, this condition often runs in families. It is not necessarily more common in children with ASD. It seems to get worse in teenage years, perhaps because of hormonal effects. Another reason it may get worse in adolescence is that teens tend to stay up late to complete homework or to chat with their friends.

Morning light can help "correct the biological clock" and "advance" sleep phase, making it easier for the child to fall asleep at night. Sometimes a light box, which emits bright light, is used in the winter months. Children can sit in front of the light box as they get ready for school or wear a light visor to get their morning dose of bright light. It is important to check with your child's health care professional before using these devices, however, as light can have side effects and affect a child's mood.

Anxiety

Many children and teens with and without ASD are anxious from time to time. Like Jennifer in the story above, they may worry about monsters when they are young and social situations (as at school) when they are older. This kind of anxiety is not considered a medical problem as long as it does not affect the child's ability to function at home or school.

Anxiety becomes a medical concern if the child's ability to function at home or at school is affected. Children with ASD are more likely to experience anxiety disorders than other children. The good news is that anxiety is highly treatable.

As mentioned in the story of Jennifer at the start of the chapter, one way of treating anxiety is with cognitive behavioral therapy (CBT). This involves having the child learn to manage their fears (the cognitive part) and also learn ways to relax (the behavioral part). Medications may also be prescribed to reduce anxiety. Some of these medications may have side effects, including some that can affect sleep, so it is important to carefully discuss the pros and cons of medication with your child's health care professional.

Sleep Apnea

Sleep apnea is a condition in which a person stops breathing periodically during sleep for at least two breath cycles, although pauses in breathing can last for many seconds. The episodes of apnea (breathing cessation) are caused by a problem in the brain in the case of central sleep apnea or by an obstruction in the airway (such as enlarged tonsils) in the case of obstructive apnea. Snoring is one of the major signs of sleep apnea, but noisy breathing can also be a sign. In addition, because their sleep is disrupted at night, children may be either sleepy or overly active during the day. (Unlike adults, children whose sleep is disrupted can be more active than usual!)

One risk factor for sleep apnea is having a family history of sleep apnea, since facial structures that can contribute to apnea (large tongue, small airway) often run in families. Other risk factors include being overweight or having a condition in which the facial structure is affected (e.g., Down syndrome).

If your child is suspected of having sleep apnea, an overnight sleep study can determine whether he is stopping breathing (see the section on "Preparing for a Sleep Study" below). Treatments include removing the tonsils and adenoids (two structures that can block the airway), having the child sleep on his side, helping the child lose weight, or continuous positive airway therapy (CPAP), which uses air to open up the blocked airway, thereby relieving the blockage.

Narcolepsy

Narcolepsy is a brain condition which causes excessive sleepiness during the day. While the cause is still being explored, it is likely the result of a shortage of hypocretin, a brain chemical that promotes wakefulness. One theory is that the body's immune system mistakenly attacks hypocretin-containing brain cells in the hypothalamus, a part of the brain that controls wake and sleep.

Other symptoms of narcolepsy are related to experiencing rapid-eye-movement sleep (dream sleep) at times when we don't normally experience this type of sleep. Symptoms may include:

- vivid dreams,
- feeling paralyzed (unable to move muscles) when falling asleep or waking up,
- sleep-related hallucinations (seeing or hearing things that are not actually present, as if in a dream) when falling asleep or waking up, or
- cataplexy (losing muscle tone and falling to the ground or dropping objects from the hand) during times of strong emotion or excitement.

These other symptoms may not be present, however, and sleepiness may be the only symptom. Narcolepsy is diagnosed by a careful clinical history combined with an overnight sleep study (to exclude other causes of sleepiness, such as sleep apnea). A daytime study is also done to measure how long it takes for the child to fall asleep and whether he quickly goes into rapid-eye-movement sleep (which is one of the symptoms of narcolepsy). Narcolepsy is treated with medications that improve alertness and decrease symptoms such as cataplexy.

Restless Legs Syndrome (RLS)

Restless Legs Syndrome (RLS) is a condition in which children have discomfort in their legs, along with an urge to move them. The discomfort has been described in many ways, including creeping, itching, crawling, and tingling, although it is often difficult for a child with ASD to describe these symptoms. Symptoms are usually worse at night and when sitting or lying down, and may be helped by moving the legs or having the legs rubbed. A child with RLS symptoms may also have lots of movement during sleep or tangled bedsheets. Parents may describe sleep as "restless."

When RLS interferes with a child being able to fall asleep or stay asleep, the sleep disruption may result in daytime sleepiness or behavior problems such as irritability, moodiness, inattention, or hyperactivity. Children who express symptoms of RLS (e.g., say they have creeping, itching, crawling, or tingling feelings), or who otherwise show symptoms (e.g., ask to have their legs rubbed at bedtime, especially if they also have restless sleep) should have their blood ferritin level checked. The ferritin level is a blood test that measures how much iron is stored in the body; low iron stores have been linked to RLS symptoms.

It is not known whether RLS is more common in children with ASD, but children with ASD may be more at risk for RLS due to being picky eaters or being on special diets that don't provide enough iron. Even if the ferritin level is normal (usually above 10-20 nanograms per milliliter (ng/ml) of blood), if it is below 50 ng/ml in someone with RLS, many experts recommend taking an iron supplement. In addition to ferritin, certain medications can help RLS symptoms.

Tooth Grinding (Bruxism)

Tooth grinding, also called bruxism, is a condition in which children grind and clench their teeth. It can happen during the day or night. The cause is not clear, although anxiety or stress can play a role. Tooth grinding may also occur because the top and bottom teeth aren't aligned properly, or as a response to pain (such as an earache). It is not known if children with ASD have more bruxism than those who are typically developing.

When tooth grinding occurs on a regular basis, the teeth can become worn down and flattened. Children may develop jaw pain, headaches, or ear aches. The treatment for tooth grinding is to wear a mouth guard that protects the teeth. Dentists can confirm signs of tooth grinding and fit children with mouth guards.

Preparing for a Sleep Study

If there are suspicions that your child has sleep apnea, a sleep study can determine whether he actually stops breathing during sleep. It can also determine whether the periods of apnea occur frequently enough, and result in a low enough level of oxygen in his bloodstream, that treatment is warranted.

During a sleep study, your child will need to stay overnight in a hospital or freestanding sleep lab. He will have a number of electrodes (sensors) attached to his scalp, chest, and legs so that his respiration, vital signs, leg movements, etc. can be monitored during sleep. He will then be expected to sleep long enough that a clear picture emerges of what happens when he sleeps. Specifically, the evaluation will show whether and how often he stops breathing, as well as how much time he moves and spends in the different phases of sleep. During an overnight sleep study, an overnight EEG is also done at the same time. The overnight EEG can look for nighttime seizure activity.

Sleep studies are not painful, and you should be able to spend the night with your child in a separate bed. Some children, however, may be upset at having electrodes attached with slimy gel. Some children may also have difficulty sleeping in a new room with many wires attached to their bodies.

If your child needs a sleep study, there are steps you can take to help make the procedure go smoothly. Find out if you can visit the sleep lab. You might want to visit first on your own and then go another time with your child. You can write a story to help your child know what will happen. If the hospital or sleep center will allow you to do so, you might even want to take pictures of some of the equipment so that your child can see the types of materials that will be used. You can add these photos to your story.

Here are the typical steps in a sleep study:

- ✔ Check child's height and weight.
- ✔ Check blood pressure.
- ✔ Check temperature.
- ✔ Put on pajamas and get ready for bed.
- ✔ Measure child's head size with a tape measure.
- ✔ Mark areas for electrodes with a marker.
- ✔ Wash head with cleaning gel and Q-tip.
- ✔ Place electrodes on child's head and face with gel and tape.
- ✔ Wrap child's head with gauze.
- ✔ Place hat over the child's head.
- ✔ Place sensor on chest.
- ✔ Put belts on child's chest and stomach.

- ✔ Place sensors on both of child's legs.
- ✔ Place sensors on child's fingers or toes.
- ✔ Place nasal cannula under child's nose.
- ✔ Put a sensor over the cannula.
- ✔ Child goes to sleep.

Make sure your child knows that you can stay with him all night. Older children and teens may like to learn why each step is happening and what the sensors measure. For example, you can explain that the sensor on your child's chest will provide information about his heart rate during the night. The sensors on his legs will tell people if he moves his legs a lot while he is sleeping. Think about the types of words you use to describe the steps. Some children like to know the exact terms and technical details of what is happening. Other children might do better with simple explanations using familiar words. We will talk more about how to use visual schedules in Chapter 6.

Distracting and Comforting Your Child: As you can see, there are a lot of steps! Getting ready for a sleep study takes about thirty minutes. Distracting your child during the set-up makes a big difference. Check to see if you can bring your child's favorite movie, video game, or other activity that will make it easier for him to sit quietly during preparations. You might try to save some of these fun activities for the night of the study. Your child might be even more interested in his favorite movie if he hasn't watched it for a few days! The same may be true for an electronic game.

Bring comfort objects that your child uses at bedtime. Stuffed animals, special blankets, and favorite toys might make him feel more at ease. Some children will also be distracted by cause-and-effect toys; bubbles (if they are allowed in the lab); toys or books that make noises; toys that make sounds, music, or lights; and oil and water toys. If your child enjoys and is calmed by certain music, it might help to play this music while he is being prepared for the study. Fidget toys can be a fun way to give your child something to do with his hands during this time. To help your child track how long the different steps take, you might also use a variety of interesting timers, such as timers that use sand or water and oil to show how much time has passed.

You might also want to make a visual schedule for your child so that he can keep track of each stage. He may feel less anxious if he knows what will come next and what is expected of him during the time he is being prepared for the study.

As your child completes each step, praise him and let him know what a good job he is doing. You might consider giving him some small rewards for completing each step. If your child has special interests, you might try rewarding him with some stickers that reflect these interests. You can save these special stickers for the night of the sleep study so that they are more interesting and motivating for your child.

Customizing the Procedure for Your Child: Sometimes the steps of the study can be changed a little to help things go more smoothly. It might help to start with steps that are easier for your child and end with the steps that are hardest. Or it may help to give him some choices during the preparation. For example, he might be able to choose who holds some materials (you, the technician, or him), if he can watch while sensors are placed on his head, or whether he wants to sit on a chair or in your lap. You can also provide choices about rewards. For instance, offer a selection of stickers and have your child choose which one he will earn for having another sensor placed on his head. Some children become focused on choosing stickers and feel less anxious about the actual procedure. Some children do better if they can sit on a chair or on your lap instead of lying down on the bed.

Check with the people working in the sleep lab to see how flexible they are about how things are done. Your child will do best if you can talk with people in advance about what will happen and how you and the technicians can work together to make this a positive experience. Do your best to stay calm and relaxed during the procedure, since this will also help your child feel less worried. Many of the ideas we discuss in this section are from an excellent article by Elizabeth Zaremba and her colleagues.[1]

Desensitization: Some children may need extra help to prepare for a sleep study. They may need to gradually get used to some of the sleep study steps. This is called desensitization and means helping your child become less sensitive to what is done during the study. You and your child can practice some of the steps and help him get used to them a little at a time.

Desensitization works best when you take very small steps and go slowly. For example, if your child has trouble letting someone touch his head, he might need to gradually learn to allow someone to quickly touch his head for just a few seconds. You would gradually increase the amount of pressure you apply as well as the length of time you touch his head. Your child would receive rewards for each small step he takes toward accepting this procedure. You might also provide distractions for him while you are practicing each step. You could also show your child the steps by practicing with a doll and then have your child practice with the doll. Eventually, your child would be able to tolerate having sensors put on his head.

Talk with your health care provider if you think your child will need this type of help. He or she might be able to recommend a specialist who can help provide desensitization for your child or might be able to guide you through some steps to take at home with your child. He or she might also have some sample supplies used in sleep studies that your child could handle beforehand to help him feel more comfortable with the procedure.

Medications and Sleep Aids

Some parents wonder why their child can't simply be prescribed a medication to help him sleep better. After all, adults sometimes use medications themselves when they are having trouble sleeping. Medications may have side effects, however. Also, as you will learn, children who learn how to fall asleep on their own without medications may be more apt to go back to sleep on their own if they wake up during the night. For these reasons, we generally wait to use medications and try educational strategies first, as described in this book. However, there are times when a medication may be useful to use. This is a choice for you to make with your health care provider. Remember that if a medication is used, it is usually most effective if combined with educational strategies.

Melatonin is sometimes used to promote sleep in children with ASD who have difficulty falling asleep or staying asleep. Melatonin is a naturally occurring hormone that signals to the brain when it is time for sleep. It is important to check with your child's health care provider to ensure it is safe to give your child. Melatonin can interfere with other medications children are receiving. It is also important for your child's health care provider to rule out other medical causes that affect sleep, such as those discussed above (sleep apnea, parasomnias, and seizures). There are many different brands of melatonin, and you will want to make sure you use a reputable brand.

For children with ASD, melatonin is usually given thirty minutes before bedtime. The exception is for children with delayed sleep phase syndrome. Because the goal for these children is to change the timing of sleep, melatonin works best when given several hours before bedtime.

References

1. Zaremba, E. K., M. E. Barkey, C. Mesa, K. Sanniti, and C. L. Rosen, "Making Polysomnography More 'Child Friendly': A Family-Centered Care Approach." *Journal of Clinical Sleep Medicine* 1, no. 2 (April 15, 2005):189–98.

Chapter 6

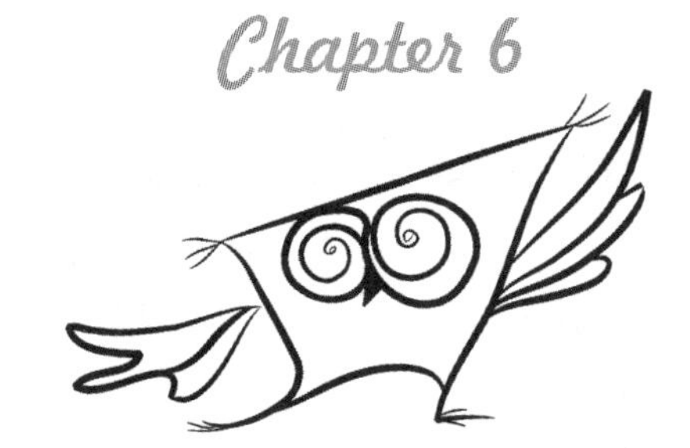

Getting Ready for Bed

Things Can Get Better!

Improving Your Child's Sleep Habits

In Chapter 4 we reviewed the questions you should try to answer when evaluating your child's sleep habits. Now it is time to talk about ways to improve your child's sleep. As we discuss these ideas, please remember that you do not need to try all of these ideas at once. It may be easier, and you may even have more success, if you start with one or two strategies and then add other changes over time. Also, please keep in mind that we are often discussing the ideal situation to promote sleep. Not all families will be able to try all of these techniques. Start with the ideas that seem easiest, and don't become discouraged if you cannot put all the steps of a plan into place all at once. Even small changes may bring promising results.

There are a number of ingredients that come together to promote good sleep. Let's start by considering all the things you can do to help your child fall asleep better before you say good night:

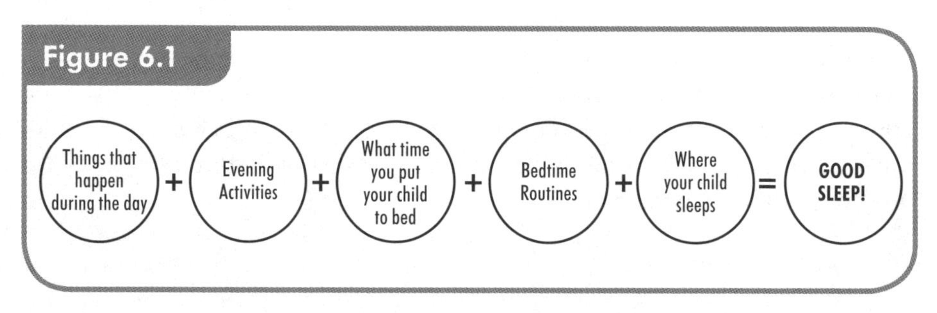

Daytime Activities Make a Difference!

What happens during the day has an effect on how we sleep at night. You can promote good sleep by focusing on some parts of your child's daily routine, including:

- physical activity
- light
- food
- naps
- bedroom use
- stressful events

Keep Things Moving

As discussed in Chapter 4, children need to get plenty of exercise during the day so they will sleep well at night. Many children with autism spectrum disorders are quite active. Others resist any physical activity. You may have to think creatively about ways to get your child to move more during the day. Some children enjoy yoga or dance. There are also video fitness programs and dance videos that encourage children to move.

Here's how Mia's family motivated her to get more exercise:

> *Mia liked to play with her stuffed animals in her playroom. She would sit quietly, and was inactive for most of the day. Her mother bought some special animal stickers for Mia. She promised Mia a sticker if she would walk with her to the end of her block. She would also get a sticker when she walked back home. Mia liked the stickers. She walked with her mother once each day for a week. Her mother slowly increased the distance Mia needed to walk to earn a sticker. Soon, Mia was walking to the park and back as part of her daily routine.*

Try to make sure that your child is not exercising too close to bedtime. Some children participate in sports and other physical activities after school. These sometimes take place later in the evening. If your child has some downtime after these events, she will be better able to unwind and be ready for sleep once she is in bed.

Bring on the Sunshine

Exposure to natural light early in the day brings down the melatonin levels we produce. We want low levels of melatonin during the day, as this increases our alertness. Open the curtains and shades and let in the sunshine first thing in the morning. Getting outside and being physically active go hand-in-hand. Your child can then meet two key goals of daytime behaviors at the same time: light exposure and exercise.

During the winter it may be difficult for your child to get the light she needs to bring down melatonin levels. Short winter days and cloudy weather can limit light, and children often spend less time outdoors when the weather is cold. As mentioned in Chapter 5, some people respond well to phototherapy or light boxes to get additional light. Check with your health care provider before using this device.

Food Matters

Children should not eat or drink foods with caffeine (according to the National Sleep Foundation; http://www.sleepfoundation.org). Caffeine may:

- ✓ interfere with sleep (studies show that the more caffeine a child eats or drinks, the less she sleeps[1])
- ✓ suppress hunger
- ✓ affect nutrition (eating or drinking foods and beverages with caffeine will take the place of eating or drinking foods with more nutrients)

As we discussed in Chapter 4, caffeine may be present in a number of different foods and drinks. Some children are sensitive to even small amounts of caffeine, and having any caffeine can have a big impact on their sleep. We suggest completely removing caffeine from your child's diet. This may be difficult, since it can be very hard to change the eating habits of children with autism spectrum disorders. There are, however, some helpful strategies to reduce caffeine in your child's diet, especially in beverages.

First, try using a caffeine-free version of your child's drink. Some soft drinks or sodas have both caffeinated and decaffeinated versions. Second, you might be able to gradually "water down" the caffeinated soda with another drink. One trick is to do this so gradually that it is very hard to notice any difference. Try substituting one-sixteenth of a cup of a non-caffeinated drink for the same amount of the caffeinated beverage. Water or a drink without caffeine that is similar to your child's beverage might be a good choice. After a few days of using one-sixteenth of a cup of the non-caffeinated liquid, try substituting one-eighth of a cup.

Some children with autism spectrum disorders have very sensitive senses of taste. They can notice even the smallest difference in their foods. It is hard to change their foods or drinks. For these children, it may work to gradually decrease the amount of drink with caffeine that they can have at any given time.

While the goal would ideally be to remove all foods with caffeine, some compromise may be required. This is especially true for older children and teens. Many popular drinks for teens have a large amount of caffeine. Educate your teen about the effects of caffeine and consider developing some rules together. For example, you might decide to limit caffeine after 12:00 p.m. in the afternoon. You might also choose to review the guidelines we discussed in Chapter 4 with your teen and use these to decide how much caffeine she should have in a day. Think, too, about whether your child is taking any medications that have caffeine. If this is the case, consider talking with your child's health care provider about whether this might be affecting her ability to fall asleep at night.

Naps Can Be Tricky

Children differ in their need for naps, although many toddlers and preschoolers do need them. How do you know whether your child still needs a nap? Parents quickly learn that a nap is still required on a day when a child misses one! Some children outgrow the need for naps sooner than others. There can be some hard transitions when children need a nap some days and don't need one another day.

Some young children can fall asleep better at night if they haven't had a nap during the day. Here's an example of how this can work: Ernesto sleeps a total of ten hours a day. He goes to sleep at 10:00 p.m. and wakes up at 6:00 a.m. He naps for two hours in the afternoon, and sleeps for eight hours at night. His parents would like him to go to bed earlier in the evening. They notice that he seems fine on days when he does not nap. So, they keep him up in the afternoon and early evening. He falls asleep at 8:00 p.m. and sleeps until 6:00 a.m. He still gets ten hours of sleep. This seems to be the right amount of sleep for him. His sleep is now combined into a single night's sleep.

We recommend ending naps by 4:00 p.m. at the latest. Naps that go later than that will get in the way of your child falling asleep at night. We have found that some teens really need to take a nap. As they move into the teenage years, children develop a later sleep schedule. Since they are often required to get up very early, they are often tired during the day. A short nap can be refreshing for some teenagers, but it is still best to avoid late afternoon naps. We would encourage teens to take a short nap (no longer than forty-five minutes), since short naps are less likely to get in the way of good sleep at night.

Beds Are for Sleep

Bedrooms should just be for sleeping. It's important to build strong connections between the bedroom and sleep. Children are more likely to fall asleep easily if the only thing they do in their bedroom is go to sleep. If they play in their rooms during the day, it is harder for them to learn that they shouldn't keep playing at bedtime.

It is best if reading, watching television, doing homework, building with blocks, or playing video games all happen in other rooms. Of course, not all families have other rooms for these activities. Still, a child's bed should definitely be just for sleeping. You can mark off play areas with tape, a small rug, or pieces of carpeting. Toys and books can be kept in bins that can be covered at night when everyone (even toys!) goes to sleep. You might also consider taking these objects out of the room at bedtime.

We recommend removing all televisions, cell phones, computers, and electronic games from the bedroom. Some children will not like these changes. If your child is used to having her television on at bedtime, you can gradually decrease the volume and brightness of the television each evening. Bear in mind that it is easier to make small changes than to change everything all at once. You can meet your child halfway. Here are some examples of ways to compromise with your child about moving the television set out of her bedroom:

- You can allow your child to watch television longer if her television isn't in her room.
- You can exchange the television for something else she really wants.
- She can go to bed later if her television is no longer in her room.
- She can cover her television with a blanket at bedtime.
- She can keep her television in her room if it is turned away from her and toward the wall at bedtime.
- She can watch television in the morning before school if she gets up early enough.

We have worked with some children who have been happy to have a small pet (such as a turtle or fish) rather than a television in their bedroom. The cage or tank goes right where the television used to be! Be careful not to get a nocturnal animal such as a pet mouse that might make noise at night. These same ideas can work when you are trying to move computers or electronic games out of the bedroom.

Try to avoid using your child's bedroom for time-outs and punishment. Otherwise, she may have negative feelings about her bedroom, which could make it harder for her to fall asleep at night. If possible, try to find another place to discipline your child so that the bedroom remains a positive space that is just for sleeping.

Another benefit of teaching your child that her bedroom is just for sleep is that you are helping her understand the difference between daytime activities and nighttime activities. Playing with toys and watching television are daytime activities. If your child likes to stay in her pajamas during the day, try to have her change into daytime clothing when she wakes up in the morning. Then, when it is time for bed, changing into pajamas will give her another clue that it is time for bed. For young children who are not yet in preschool, this may help give some structure to the day. Older children might benefit from this routine on the weekends and vacation days when regular weekday schedules have changed.

Stressful Days, Sleepless Nights

Sometimes the strain of the day makes it hard for children to fall asleep. Children with ASD are prone to feeling anxious. It can be hard for them to let go of these feelings and to relax. In particular, they often have sleep difficulties when dealing with transitions (such as the beginning or ending of the school year). While these stressful situations are often temporary, it sometimes pays to consider what can be done during the day to reduce stress and thus improve a child's ability to fall asleep at night. Here is an example:

Joseph was in second grade. He was a good sleeper, but he started to have trouble falling asleep at night. His mother did not know that his teacher had started talking to the class about moving up to third grade. She was puzzled about his sleeping difficulties. Joseph was not able to voice his concerns to his mother. During a teacher conference, she learned that Joseph was refusing to complete some of his math assignments. This was puzzling because he liked math and was good at it.

As Joseph's mother and his teacher talked, they realized that Joseph was worried about leaving second grade and his beloved teacher. They started working with him so that he could learn about what he would be doing in third grade. He visited his new teacher and was able to see some of the classroom materials. He began to feel better about third grade and started sleeping better at night.

Routine events can also make children with ASD feel anxious. Tests, school trips, assemblies, and other regular school activities may make some children worried or upset. Other children may have specific fears or phobias that upset them throughout the day. Relaxation techniques such as deep breathing, yoga, and visualization help some children. Cognitive behavioral therapy is a highly effective intervention technique that can help children master their fears and anxiety. If your child is very anxious, and if her anxiety is interfering with her day-to-day functioning, you might consider seeking assistance from a therapist trained in these techniques. We have listed some books that address anxiety in children at the end of this chapter.

What Happens in the Evening Makes a Difference:

The hour or so before bedtime can be a good time to prepare children to get a good night's sleep. The following are common factors that can affect your child's sleep: evening activities, light exposure, and routines.

Evening Activities—Do's and Don'ts

There is often a lot to be done toward the end of the day, and there may be many tasks that need to be completed to prepare for a new day. Chores need to be finished and homework may need to be completed. Many families are so busy that they forget to relax at the end of the day!

Activities to Avoid: Unwinding and settling down should be a part of the evening routine. Children sleep better when they have had an hour or so to relax before bedtime. This means being done with difficult or stimulating activities. These might include playing sports, doing homework, listening to loud music, playing stimulating computer games, or watching something exciting on television. Roughhousing and energetic activities before bed make it harder to fall asleep. Be sure to avoid anything that involves lots of physical activity. While it might seem like running and jumping would tire your child out and make her ready for sleep, the opposite is true! Lots of excitement makes it harder to wind down and relax.

Soothing Activities: Try to find some soothing activities that your child can participate in before bedtime. Some examples include listening to music, reading, drawing, or playing with certain toys. Talk with your child or teen about what will work best, and develop a list of things that will help her feel calm and settled before bed. Feeling stressed makes it hard to fall asleep, so try to avoid discussing challenging topics too close to bedtime. If your child needs to talk about stressful events, try to do this earlier in the evening, whenever possible.

Relaxation Techniques: We recommend teaching your child how to relax. These techniques can be a lifelong skill that children can use in many situations. Try teaching your child these techniques and having her practice during the day when she is calm and happy. She can then use these strategies at other times when she might need them.

Young children can learn some simple strategies to relax. For example, they can learn to take a deep breath, hold it in, and then let it out slowly. You can help them practice this by teaching them to "blow out the candles." You can then use this phrase to help them breathe in a relaxing way. Some children also respond well to the phrase "smell the flowers" in much the same way.

Older children and teens can learn how to tense and relax their entire bodies. One way to do this is to tense and relax different parts of the body one by one. Here is an example of one way to do this:

- Squeeze your eyes shut tight and then open them slowly.
- Wrinkle your nose as if something smells bad then let go.
- Put your teeth together and clench them and then let your mouth go slack.
- Stretch your left arm out in front of you and then let it drop.
- Stretch your right arm out in front of you and then let it drop.
- Make a fist with your left hand and then let go.
- Make a fist with your right hand and then let go.
- Tighten up your stomach muscles and gradually let them relax.
- Push your toes down into the ground then let them go loose.
- Let your whole body go limp. Pretend you are a ragdoll or a floppy stuffed animal.

You can guide your child through this process by telling her what to do using a reassuring and positive tone. While she will be tensing her muscles, the process should not hurt or be uncomfortable. Some children might need reminders not to squeeze too tightly.

Your child might also benefit from guided imagery strategies. These involve visualizing a pleasant place (such as a beach or a meadow) and imagining the different sensations (such as sounds, smells, and special images) associated with this location. We have included references to some books that provide detailed information about relaxation techniques at the end of this chapter.

Sensory techniques can also be very calming. Some examples of potentially calming sensory activities include rocking, swinging, swaddling, deep pressure, massage, and joint compression. Some relaxing yoga positions may also be beneficial. Children have different responses to different techniques, and what is calming for one child may be exciting for another. It is often a matter of trial and error to find the right sensory techniques that will work for your child.

Bedtime Snacks: Some children benefit from having a light snack before bed. Remember, however, that heavy meals and spicy food may interfere with sleep. A small snack before bed will keep your child from being hungry during the night. Good choices for bedtime snacks include a small serving of cereal, milk, cheese, crackers, yogurt, or bananas.

Warm Baths: A warm bath or shower before bed can also be relaxing and lead to better sleep. This will, of course, depend on your child's response to bath time. If bath time is very exciting and stimulating for your child, it would not be a good idea to have bath time too close to bed time.

While many children with ASD find bath time to be relaxing, they often dislike having their hair washed. They may be especially sensitive to having water on their heads. If this is the case for your child, you might eliminate hair washing from her bath-time routine at bedtime. You might try to save hair washing for a weekend morning. You can also try a gentle approach to hair washing. Instead of pouring water over your child's head to remove shampoo, try using a wet washcloth. Make sure the washcloth is not too wet. This method takes longer than using a cup for rinsing, but it does the trick and often saves lots of tears and distress.

Some children also have trouble when it is time to come out of their bath. It is a relaxing experience until it is time to stop, but then they might get very upset. It often helps to use a timer so that your child can see when bath time will be over. It also can help to have a fun (and relaxing) activity follow bath time.

Light: Consider the Source!

It is best to turn the lights down low about an hour before bed. This can often be difficult, but try to do the best you can. Dimmer switches can be used to dim the lights in the evening. You might also consider using black-out curtains if you need to block the light from cars, neighboring homes, or streetlights. Just remember to open the curtains in the morning to let in the sunlight.

You also need to be aware of light from other sources such as televisions, computers, smart phones, and electronic media and games. The bluish light that is emitted from screens of many smart phones, computers, and fluorescent light bulbs may interfere with melatonin production and sleep. Older children and teens often spend a great deal of time on the computer late into the night.

Some parents develop contracts with their teens about computer use in the evening. They may set limits on using the Internet and the computer and even write up contracts spelling out the limits. If your child honors the contract, she can earn rewards, which might include extra computer time on the weekends. Some parents unplug all gadgets at a specific time, put computers on a timer, or install software that limits computer use.

Turning electronics off before bedtime might be particularly hard for a teen who does not want to put away her smart phone. You may need to negotiate with your teen about this and provide some incentives to help her stick to an agreed-upon schedule. Helping your teen understand the reasons and benefits of good sleep may help. You might consider trying to set a good example by turning off your own smart phone and other electronic devices before bedtime!

Evening Habits

If possible, develop a regular routine in the evening, and try to do things in the same order. You might try turning down the lights at the same time each evening and engaging in some of the same calm activities in the same sequence each night. Turning down the lights about an hour before it is time to start a bedtime routine promotes good sleep. If some activities are harder for your child, try to do them earlier in the evening rather than right before you start your child's bedtime routine.

Bedtime Routines

After evening activities are done, it is time to get ready for bed. Your child should go through the same bedtime routine each night. Completing the same activities each night before bed lets us know it is time for bed. Our bodies become more ready for sleep if we follow the same routine. If a child brushes her teeth each night at the same time before going to bed, her body recognizes that it is time to get ready to fall asleep during tooth brushing time.

Use Visual Supports

Many children with autism spectrum disorders benefit from the use of visual aids. These might include pictures or objects that you use to teach your child about her day and let her know what to expect. Use of these tools takes advantage of the strong visual interests and preference for sameness that many children with ASD have.

Benefits of Visual Supports: We suggest using visual supports to teach your child about her bedtime routine. This will help her know what to expect at bedtime, and she will be able to see each step of her routine. Providing your

Ideas for creating a good bedtime routine:

★ Use visual aids.
★ Pick just a few activities (between three and six).
★ Try to make sure each activity is easy and relaxing.
★ Put the hardest or most exciting activities earlier in the schedule.
★ Arrange activities so that your child is moving toward her room.
★ Keep the routine short.
★ Follow the same routine each night.
★ Use the same visual supports every night.
★ Provide nonverbal cues that it is time for bed.
★ Use the same verbal cue each time you tell your child to use her schedule.
★ Let your child be in charge of using the schedule (with help from you as needed).
★ Reward your child for using her schedule!

child with a visual schedule allows her to see what activity she should be doing and what will come next. Most children feel less anxious when they know what will happen next, and being calm at bedtime will lead to better sleep.

Transitions may be particularly hard for children with ASD, and making the shift from being awake to going to bed is often a difficult transition for many children with and without ASD. Visual aids may help with that transition and allow your child to focus on bedtime activities. They give children another way to understand what they need to do, and this can help when words alone don't seem to be enough. A visual schedule can also be rewarding to use. Many adults have their own checklists of tasks. It feels good to cross off something on your "to do" list, and children enjoy doing this as well. We feel good about ourselves and the tasks we have finished.

Visual schedules may also decrease power struggles between you and your child. When your child is following a visual schedule, you don't need to tell her what to do during each step of her bedtime routine. It lessens the chances that your child will forget or be confused about the steps in her routine. She is much more likely to follow the routine and less likely to refuse your requests. Using a visual schedule will also help you remember to follow a consistent bedtime routine and will allow others to guide your child through her routine when you can't be present.

Making Visual Schedules: Decide on what types of materials you will use to make a visual schedule for your child. You might use photographs, drawings, cartoons, or pictures. Some older children and teens prefer written checklists. You can put the written lists on a dry erase board or a chalkboard, or you can laminate a piece of cardboard that lists each step. Children can then cross off or erase each step as it is completed. Some children use objects instead of pictures.

An example of a visual schedule is presented in Figure 6.2. We have also included some pictures you can use for your schedules in Appendix F. These visual support materials were developed by Vanderbilt Kennedy Center's Treatment and Research Institute for Autism Spectrum Disorders (kc.vanderbilt.edu/triad) and may also be found in the Autism Treatment Network/Autism Intervention Research Network on Physical Health (ATN/AIR-P) *Sleep Booklet-Parent Booklet and Quick Tips* (http://www.autismspeaks.org/science/resources-programs/autism-treatment-network/tools-you-can-use/sleep-tool-kit).[2] This resource and a variety of other tool kits (including one on using visual supports) are available free of charge from the ATN/AIR-P. They can be downloaded at http://www.autismspeaks.org/family-services/tool-kits.

When you make your schedule, you might want to put your pictures on cardboard and then cover them with contact paper or laminate them so that they will last longer. You can put Velcro or magnets on the back of each picture. Children often enjoy pulling the pictures of each activity off of their charts. You can put the pictures on a strip of cardboard or a magnet board. There are many ways you can get pictures for schedules:

- You (or your child) can draw them.
- You can take photographs of objects.
- You can buy or download photos of objects; a good website for photos is "Picture This" (www.silverliningmm.com).
- Take photographs of your child doing a routine (such as brushing her teeth).
- You can download or print out line drawings from sources such as:
    - Do2Learn: http://www.do2learn.com/picturecards/printcards/
    - Kid Access: www.kidaccess.com
- You can cut out pictures from magazines.
- You can use programs that make line drawings (such as Mayer-Johnson's Boardmaker program at www.mayerjohnson.com).

If you don't think your child will understand a schedule that uses pictures, try using real objects. You can use a set of boxes and put one object for each activity in each box. Let's say that your child's bedtime routine includes brushing teeth, drinking some water, using the toilet, reading a book, and a massage with lotion. You can set up some boxes containing the following items in a place near her bedroom: a toothbrush, a special cup that is used just for a bedtime drink, a roll of toilet paper, her bedtime book, and a bottle of lotion that is only used for her bedtime massage. Your child would take each object out of the box and use it when it is time for that part of her bedtime routine. You might also save a special object that is just used for bedtime. This might be a small blanket, pillow, or stuffed animal. Once your child has this object, she should get into her bed.

Even if you don't use a set of visual supports for your child, write down her schedule so that you are keeping a consistent routine each night. Use the same words each night to label what you are doing.

Figure 6.2—Visual Schedule Example

Brush teeth
Draw
Get a drink
Lotion
Hug & kiss goodnight
Go to bed

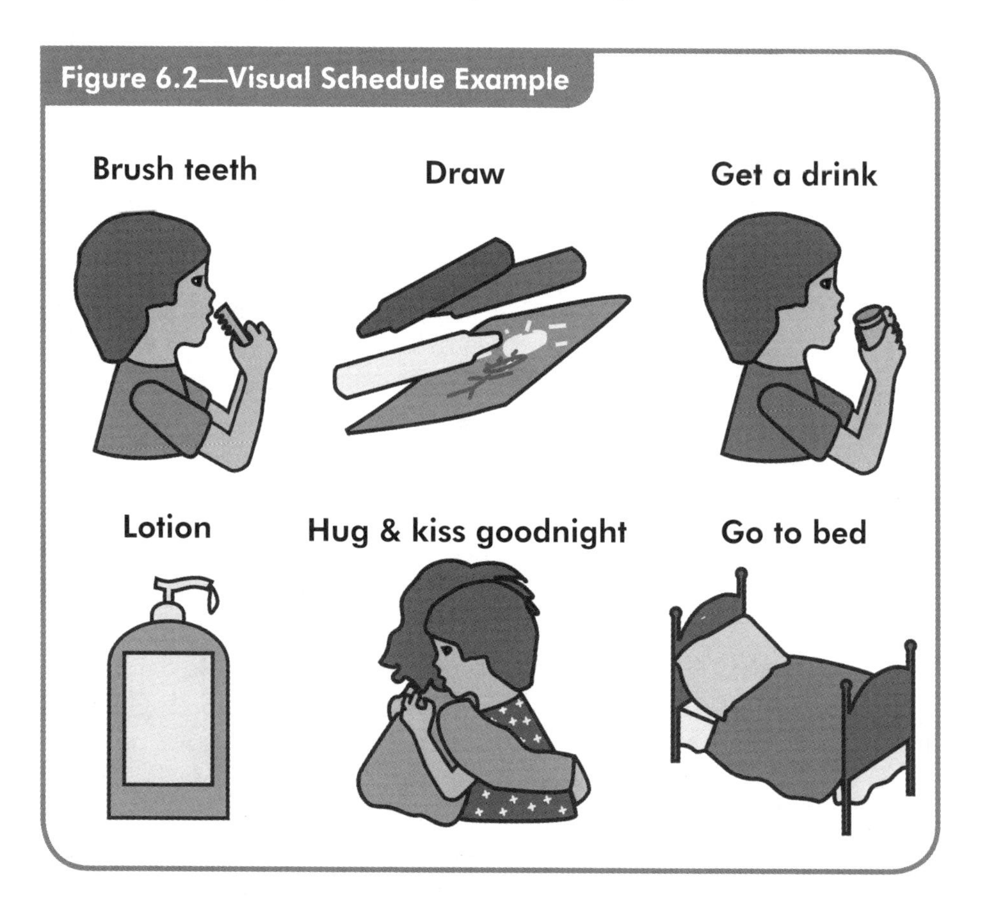

Carefully Choose and Sequence Activities in the Routine

Pick Just a Few Activities: Bedtime schedules should involve a small number of tasks. We suggest somewhere between three and six. If there are too few activities, your child's schedule may not provide enough structure for her. If there are too many, it may be hard for your child to link these activities with feeling sleepy.

Make Sure Each Activity Is Easy and Relaxing: You want your child to be in a calm state before bed. Hard activities may make her frustrated and upset. Exciting activities may get her too energized to go to sleep. Be sure to end the bedtime routine with activities that promote good sleep.

Put Hard or Stimulating Activities Earlier in the Schedule: Sometimes a bedtime activity will be difficult. For example, brushing teeth is often very challenging for children with ASD. Since your child must brush her teeth before going to bed, you need to think about when she should do it. Try to make this the first activity in your child's bedtime routine. If it is really hard for her, you might want to do this earlier in the evening when you know your child is done eating for the night. That way it doesn't even need to be part of her bedtime routine. Hair washing can also be hard. Sometimes it is better to do this in the morning or when your child first gets home from school. Try not to have one difficult routine directly follow another. Bedtime can be more pleasant if you put easy routines after hard routines. Have your child complete a fun and relaxing activity after completing a hard one. For example, if brushing teeth is difficult for your child and reading a book is calming, it might help to have a schedule in which reading a favorite book always follows tooth brushing. Your child would always move on to reading even if she really struggles during tooth brushing.

Arrange Activities So Your Child Moves toward the Bedroom: Try to set up bedtime routines so that you finish in your child's bedroom. For example, start with tasks that happen in the living room, move to the bathroom, and finish in the bedroom. Put your child's visual schedule in a central place in the house. Make sure she can reach the schedule, and keep it in the same place every night.

Keep the Routine Short: An effective bedtime routine lasts fifteen to thirty minutes. Bedtime routines often get longer as children get older. We might expect very young children to have a bedtime routine that only lasts about fifteen minutes. Although older children tend to have longer bedtime routines, it is best if a routine does not last more than sixty minutes.

Follow the Same Routine Each Night: Keep things consistent. Use the same pictures or objects each night. This will make it easier for your child to learn the routine. She will be more relaxed and ready for sleep.

Use the Schedule

Teach Your Child to Use Her Schedule: If your child has never used a visual schedule, you will need to teach her how. Spend some time showing her how it works. She may need some prompts to use it. Use as few words as possible. It is easier to slowly stop using physical prompts than verbal prompts. The goal is to have children use their schedules on their own. When you use physical prompts, stand behind your child and prompt her by moving her arm or gently tapping her elbow to take the card off her schedule. Your child will learn how to use her schedule more quickly if she doesn't rely on your facial expressions or other cues to help her understand what you want her to do.

Teach Your Child When to Use Her Schedule: Use the same cue every night to let your child know it is time to use her schedule. This might be a nonverbal sign. You can also use certain words. Some examples include: "look at your plan," "check your list," "time for bed," and "what's next?"

Make Sure Your Child Takes Care of Her Own Schedule: Your child should be taking cards off her schedule or checking things off her list. If she needs help, you can guide her hand to do this. Use a hand-over-hand prompt if you need to.

Give Your Child a Reward: You may give your child some small prizes such as stickers, as well as praise and hugs while she is following her schedule. You can give her rewards after she finishes each task or after she has finished her whole schedule.

Visual schedules make change easier. A visual schedule at bedtime addresses a major change in the day that can be very difficult: the change from being awake to going to bed. We strongly encourage you to use a visual schedule at bedtime. Even if you are not sure it will work, give it a try! It can make bedtime go a lot more smoothly.

Provide Nonverbal Cues That It Is Time for Bed

Many of the ideas in this book apply to all children with autism spectrum disorders. We have found, however, that children with limited verbal skills often benefit from some additional strategies. These techniques work for children with fluent speech, but they can provide extra support for children who use few, if any, words.

You need to give your child many signals that it is time to go to sleep. Providing the same set of sensory events each night can teach children it is time for bed. Think about your child's responses to different sensations and add sensory-based strategies that are calm and comforting to her routine. Bearing in mind that we all respond to sensory input in different ways, here are some examples of what might work. Be sure to use each strategy in the same way and in the same order each night.

Give children many consistent environmental cues that it is time for bed. Decide on what these cues might be and then use the same cues each night at bedtime.

- rocking
- swinging
- getting a massage
- rubbing on lotion
- receiving strong hugs
- being wrapped in a blanket
- listening to music
- wearing a weighted vest
- smelling scented sprays or candles (with the lights down low—be sure to blow out the candle before your child falls asleep!)
- chewing on something (like gum, vinyl tubing, or crunchy food or chewy food)

Make a Bedtime Schedule

Use the worksheet in Table 6.1 to create a bedtime schedule for your child. We have included a number of common bedtime activities. Look at this list and see if they are part of your child's current bedtime routine. List any activities in your child's routine that we did not include. Now think about whether each activity is easy or hard for your child. Put an "E" next to activities that are easy and an "H" next to activities that are hard. It is best to only include easy activities in a bedtime routine. If an activity is difficult for your child, try to take it out of her schedule or put it early in the bedtime routine. If your child gets upset if you read to her, that should not be part of her bedtime schedule.

Now think about whether these activities are stimulating or relaxing. Put an "S" next to activities that are stimulating and an "R" next to activities that are relaxing. Some activities might be easy but also stimulating. For instance, a child might really enjoy playing video games. This might be easy for her but also stimulating.

Once you have rated each activity, rank the activities in order of your child's preference. Remember that hard or exciting activities should occur early in a bedtime routine, if at all. You can then use this list to plan a bedtime schedule for your child. Creating a bedtime routine is something that you can do on your own, with a spouse or partner, or with your child. Think about asking your child about the plan. Your child may have some good ideas about what will work for him or her. You can talk with your child about what will work and come up with a plan together. Older children and teens will usually want to be included in this process. You will find another copy of the Bedtime Routines Worksheet in Appendix E and at www.woodbinehouse.com/SolvingSleepProblems.asp.

Table 6.1—Bedtime Routines Worksheet

Activities	Occurs	Is the activity easy (E) or hard (H)?	Is the activity stimulating (S) or relaxing (R)?	Rank in order of preference (1, 2, 3)
Taking a bath				
Washing hair				
Changing into pajamas				
Getting a drink				
Brushing teeth				
Using the bathroom				
Singing quiet songs				
Reading				
Other:				

Using the information from the Bedtime Routines Worksheet, plan a bedtime schedule for your child:

Order	Activity	Is the activity easy (E) or hard (H)?	Is the activity stimulating (S) or relaxing (R)?

Developed by the Vanderbilt Treatment and Research Institute for Autism Spectrum Disorders.

Here is an example of how one mother used the Bedtime Routines Worksheet to develop a sleep routine for her son with ASD, Ryan.

Activities	**Occurs**	**Is the activity easy (E) or hard (H)?**	**Is the activity simulating (S) or relaxing (R)?**	**Rank in order of preference (1, 2, 3)**
Taking a bath	X	E	R	7
Washing hair	X	H	S	8
Changing into pajamas	X	E	R	5
Getting a drink	X	E	R	4
Brushing teeth	X	H	S	6
Using the bathroom	X	E	R	3
Singing quiet songs				
Reading				
Other: Playing with cars	X	E	R	2
Other: Watching videos	X	E	S	1

After thinking about her son's schedule, Ryan's mother decided to let him watch videos after dinner but before his bedtime routine starts. Although he likes this activity, he gets very excited when he watches videos. In addition, his mother is concerned about the light exposure from videos and wants to decrease the amount of light Ryan is exposed to before bed. Even though watching videos is his favorite activity, she will omit it from his bedtime routine and make sure that he gets to watch videos earlier in the evening. She is also going to let him watch a video in the morning as a reward for sleeping through the night.

Ryan's mother decides to have her son start his routine by brushing his teeth. This is hard for Ryan, and he usually gets upset during this activity. He will get to play with his cars once he is done brushing his teeth. Playing with cars is one of his favorite activities and it is relaxing for him. He will get to play with his cars even if he has trouble with teeth brushing and even if he can't brush his teeth for as long as his mother would like. She knows that he will continue to improve in his area. In fact, she is gradually increasing the time that she expects him to brush his teeth, and she is helping him get used to this activity by massaging his gums before he starts to brush his teeth.

The rest of Ryan's bedtime routine will have him complete activities that bring him closer to his bedroom. After playing with his cars, he will then get a drink of water. Ryan likes his bath, but it is hard for him when his mother washes his hair. She has decided to stop washing his hair at bedtime. She will just wash his hair in the mornings on the weekends. Bedtime is her main concern right now. She would rather wash his hair less often and let him stay calm before bed. Ryan will use the bathroom after his bath and change into his pajamas. Then it will be time for bed. Here is Ryan's bedtime schedule:

Order	Activity	Is the activity easy (E) or hard (H)?	Is the activity stimulating (S) or relaxing (R)?
1	Brushing teeth	H	S
2	Playing with cars	E	R
3	Getting a drink	E	R
4	Taking a bath	E	R
5	Using the bath-room	E	R
6	Changing into pajamas	E	R

What Time Is Bedtime?

If your child is going to bed at the desired time and falls asleep about twenty minutes or so after you put her to bed, you don't need to think about changing her bedtime. You might, however, want to consider a later bedtime if she takes longer than twenty minutes to fall asleep. There are number of things to consider when finding a bedtime for your child:

- What time does your child fall asleep at night?
- When do you need your child to be in bed?
- When do other people in the family go to bed?
- Is this a good bedtime for all the days of the week?

Consider the Benefits of a Later Bedtime

Your child may be sleepier if she goes to bed later and may not struggle as much. This will lead to better sleep habits. A later bedtime also avoids the "forbidden zone" that we talked about in Chapter 1. You can try putting your child to bed at an earlier time once she has learned to fall asleep more quickly.

Choose a Time When Your Child Is Sleepy: How do you decide on a good starting time? Think about when your child actually falls asleep (not when you put her to bed). If your child is frequently falling asleep at 9:30 p.m. at night, you might pick a bedtime close to that time. If you do choose a later bedtime for your child, remember to keep her morning wake time the same. Do not let her sleep in later just because you have let her go to bed later. If she is allowed to sleep in, she may not be ready to go to sleep at her new bedtime and may still struggle with bedtime. It will also be important to avoid any naps during the day. Once good sleep habits are in place, it is often possible to move a child's bedtime to an earlier time.

Here's an example of how that might work:

Sarah's father puts her to bed at 7:30 p.m. every night. Sarah doesn't fall asleep until about 9:00 p.m., however. Sarah calls for her father, talks loudly, and asks for things such as food and drinks until she falls asleep. Sarah's father decides that Sarah is not really sleepy at 7:30. He tries putting her to bed at 8:45 instead of 7:30, and she falls asleep in about twenty minutes. He keeps her wake time the same and does not let her sleep later in the morning. Sarah's father keeps her 8:45 bedtime for a few days and notes that she is falling asleep quickly each night. After a few days, he tries putting Sarah to bed at 8:30 p.m. She still falls asleep in about twenty minutes. Every few days, he makes her bedtime about fifteen minutes earlier, and she continues to fall asleep quickly. However, when he puts her to bed at 7:45 p.m., she has a lot of trouble falling asleep. Her father now knows that an 8:00 p.m. bedtime is best for her.

Sarah's story shows that an early bedtime sometimes makes it harder to fall asleep. Sarah wasn't sleepy at 7:30 p.m. She wasn't ready for sleep, so she did other things instead of settling down for sleep. It turned out that she was sleepy and ready for bed at a later time. She then developed some new and better bedtime habits.

One way to think about the importance of avoiding the "forbidden zone" and putting your child to bed too early is to remember a night when you went to bed before your regular bedtime. Most of us can recall a time when we decided to go to bed extra early in order to be fresh and ready for an early appointment. Unless you were terribly sleep deprived, you probably did not fall asleep at the earlier bedtime, and you most likely had trouble falling asleep at your regular bedtime because of your difficulty falling asleep when you first went to bed. You may have even stayed up much later than usual because you became somewhat distressed as you tossed and turned in bed. Children who are put to bed too early may be experiencing these same feelings each night.

Choose a Time That Works for Everyone: You will want to choose a time that will work for you and the rest of the family. It may be hard to let your child with an autism spectrum disorder go to bed at a late hour. She might be going to bed later than her brothers and sisters, and they may tell you that this isn't fair. A late bedtime for your child might also make it hard for you to finish your chores or have some alone time with your spouse or partner.

You need to balance your child's needs with everyone else's needs. We certainly respect a parent's decision about what will work best for everyone in the family. Think about how much time you spend with your child at night, however, after you put her to bed at an early hour. How much time do you spend with her after you say goodnight? It might be less time-consuming, stressful, and frustrating to choose a later bedtime for your child. For example, Jessica's family decided that her 8:30 p.m. bedtime wasn't working. Jessica would cry for her parents for up to 90 minutes after they put her to bed. This was very difficult for her parents and for her older brother Nicholas.

Jessica's parents decided to put her to bed at 10:00 p.m. They wanted to help her establish good sleep habits and planned to have her go to bed earlier once some good routines were established. They had a list of quiet activities that Jessica could do on her own while she was awake, so they could finish their nighttime chores during this time. At first, Nicholas was angry that his little sister was going to bed after he did. His parents explained their plan to Nicholas. Nicholas and Jessica used to get the same amount of screen time each day, but Nicholas started getting extra screen time since he is older than Jessica. Once the plan was put in place, Jessica went to sleep without difficulty at 10:00 p.m., and Nicholas appreciated how quiet it was in the evening.

Allow Your Child Some Downtime: A later bedtime might also make it easier to give your child some downtime before she goes to bed. Most children benefit from having about an hour to relax before they go to sleep. It can be hard to get everything done and wind down when you have an early bedtime! A later bedtime can make it easier to finish up exciting or challenging activities and still have time to slow down. It also makes it easier to have the lights down low before bed. This all makes it easier for your child to fall asleep and develop good sleep habits.

Try to teach your older child or teen the reasons why you are recommending some downtime and low lights before bed. Learning about these types of issues can help children develop good sleep habits.

Be Consistent

You want to choose a bedtime that will be easy to keep the same during the week and weekend. A consistent bedtime and wake time will help your child's body develop a regular and natural pattern for sleep. It will be easier for your child to fall asleep at bedtime if she wakes up and goes to bed at the same time each day. But what if your schedule changes from day to day? Choose a bedtime that will work on your busiest evening and stick to that bedtime. It is better to keep to the same bedtime even if an earlier bedtime is possible on some days of the week.

Do the same with morning wake-up times. Try not to vary your wake-up times by more than one or two hours at the most. This may be difficult advice to follow, but a consistent wake and sleep schedule really is best for good sleep. It may help to plan for some special activities in the morning when your child wakes up. While it is tempting to let children sleep in on the weekends, this will ultimately make it harder for your child to learn good sleep practices.

There will, of course, be times when your child has a sleepover or other special activity, and at those times she will go to bed later. Sleeping in or staying up late will happen from time to time, but shouldn't be a regular occurrence.

Experiencing a big change in your sleep schedule is somewhat like traveling to another time zone. If you go somewhere that is several time zones away, it is difficult to have a good sleep routine. People who travel often are tired and have difficulty regulating their sleep. While this is fine once in a while, it would be very difficult to travel to other time zones every weekend and then have to return home for class or work on Monday mornings. Sleeping in for more than two hours on the weekends is similar to traveling cross-country. Instead of lettinng your child sleep very late in the morning, the best way to adjust for times when your child needs extra sleep is to plan for a well-timed nap. These naps should be short (no more than about thirty minutes), and should not occur too late in the day.

Since teens often have a naturally occurring later sleep and wake time, having to wake up early for school is difficult. If your teen has early morning school commitments, it is extra hard to think about having your teen wake up early on the weekend. Some communities have adopted a later start time for high school students. While this does not work for all families and schools, this might be a helpful practice for some.

Individualize Bedtime to Your Child's Needs

As your child gets older, you will need to include her in decisions about her bedtime. It is easier to just pick a bedtime for a younger child. Older children and teens will need to have some say about when they go to bed. The same principles about later bedtimes apply to older children. Children naturally go to sleep later as they grow older. It is likely that your teen will do better with a later bedtime. If possible let her have a later wake time as well. Many high schools now have a later start time in recognition of what we know about teens and their sleep schedules. Teens naturally go to bed later and wake up later.

Hopefully, your teen goes to a school that has a later morning start time. This works best for a teen's naturally occurring sleep schedule. Unfortunately, many high schools have a very early start time, which is quite difficult for teens. Even if your teen cannot sleep later during school days, try to have her get up at the same time on weekends. Sleeping in on the weekends makes it hard to develop a good sleep pattern.

Keeping a consistent wake time on the weekends is often challenging for families, especially for parents who are not early risers themselves! If, however, your teen is struggling with sleep, it may be especially important to maintain a consistent sleep schedule. Your teen will be able to fall asleep more readily if she has the same bedtime and wake time every day. She will then be more alert and less sleep-deprived. As we discussed in Chapter 2, a lack of sleep affects many aspects of daytime functioning.

How do we decide if we have chosen a good bedtime?

- ★ It is after the forbidden zone (see Chapter 1).
- ★ It is close to the time your child finally falls asleep after you put her to bed.
- ★ It can stay about the same every night.
- ★ It works for you and the rest of your family.

For teens who drive, it is critically important that your teen be well-rested. The National Sleep Foundation's website (www.sleepfoundation.org) states that sleep deprivation results in impaired driving that is comparable to that of drivers with a blood alcohol content of .08 percent (a level that is illegal for drivers in many states). Drowsy driving is also known to cause over 100,000 crashes each year.

Please note that we are not using the number of hours a child will be in bed as a guide for setting a bedtime. You do not need to try to make sure your child gets a certain amount of sleep. You should be more concerned with finding a good time for your child to easily fall asleep. Once your child has developed some good sleep habits, you can work on increasing the amount of sleep that she gets. Think about quality versus quantity. The first thing to do is to work on the quality of your child's sleep. Once your child has established good sleep habits, an increase in the amount of time she is sleeping may naturally follow.

There isn't one magic time that will work. It really is a matter of balancing all the factors that we have discussed.

Sleep Setting

Once your child has completed her bedtime routine, it is time to go to bed. Think about where your child will be sleeping. Do you want her to be in her own bedroom? Does she need to share a room with you or another family member? Does she have her own bed, or does she sleep with someone else? Do you want to change where she is sleeping now? There are no right or wrong answers to any of these questions, and you will make different plans for your child depending on the answers.

As you consider the different possibilities, it will be important to keep in mind one key concept. We'll talk more about this in Chapter 7, but the basic ideas is to make sure that whatever happens at the beginning of the night stays the same all night long. So, for example, if you want your child to sleep in her own bed during the night, she needs to fall asleep in her bed at the beginning of the night. If you let her fall asleep on the couch and then move her to her bedroom after she falls asleep, it is likely that she will wake up during the night. If she falls asleep cuddling next to someone, she will need to keep cuddling with that person throughout the night. Now, let's look at some different sleep settings for your child:

Sleeping in Her Own Room: Has your child always slept in her own room, or will she be moving back there? If she is moving back or starting to sleep in her own room for the very first time, you can prepare her for this change. You can write a story so that she understands what will be happening. There are a number of techniques that you can use to write a story that teaches a child about specific concepts. Here is a story to help a boy learn about starting to sleep in his own room:

Sleep is a good thing. Everyone needs a good night's sleep. Mommy and Daddy sleep in one room. I used to sleep with Mommy and Daddy. I am a big boy now. I am going to sleep in my own room. My room is special. I have a poster with cars on my bedroom wall. I have a bedspread with a picture of a car on it. I have a nightlight that stays on all night. Mommy and Daddy will give me a hug and say goodnight. I'll go to sleep in my own bed. When I wake up in the morning I will see Mommy and Daddy. I will get a special prize for sleeping in my room all night.

We learned how to write stories that teach children about events and experiences in their lives by reading Carol Gray's book *The New Social Story™ Book* (Arlington, TX: Future Horizons, 2010). Her website at www.thegray-center.org/social-stories also has information about this technique. Some key ideas to remember when writing a story that teaches your child an important concept include personalizing the story, adding pictures or photographs, using positive language, and writing the story from your child's perspective.

It can be fun and beneficial to have children work with their parents to decorate their rooms. They can also receive rewards for learning to sleep on their own. We discuss types of rewards in Chapter 7. Some children might need extra support to learn to sleep on their own. Chapter 7 also covers some of the things you can do to help your child learn to sleep independently.

Sharing a Room: Some children like sharing a bedroom with another person. They like the company and are less anxious than when they sleep alone. Others are distracted and have more trouble sleeping with someone else in the room. Of course, some families do not have a choice and need to have their children share a bedroom. When brothers and sisters share a bedroom, it sometimes helps to set some rules about what needs to happen at bedtime. Brothers and sisters often benefit from guidelines about when they need to stop talking. They can help each other be calm and settle in for sleep.

You might consider staggering your children's bedtimes. One child can go to bed before the other. There are fewer distractions, and it is easier for both children to fall asleep. This might also give you the opportunity to spend some special one-on-one time with each of your children.

If you share a bedroom with your child, you need to decide whether you will share the same bed. If you do share a bed, and your child cuddles with you, remember that she will need to be able to cuddle with you all night in order to remain asleep. It often works best to help your child fall asleep on her own even if you are sharing a bedroom. When parents share a bedroom with their children, they should make sure that their children are falling asleep on their own. You can have your child sleep in a bed near yours. Or if you share a bed with your child, try to put a body pillow or other divider between you and your child.

Matthew and his younger brother, Andrew, shared a bedroom and went to bed at the same time. Andrew always fell asleep right away. But Matthew was not ready for bed. He would call for his parents many times after they said goodnight. They always came right away because they didn't want Andrew to wake up. Matthew and Andrew's parents did not have enough room in the house to separate the boys. They decided to put Matthew to bed an hour later than Andrew. They explained the new plan to the boys and gave them rewards for following the plan. This later bedtime was better for Matthew, and he went to sleep much more quickly.

Sleeping in a Common Area: Some families live in small quarters. They may not have enough room in their home to allow their children to sleep in a separate location. Their children may need to sleep in the same areas where people eat and watch television. It can be challenging for children to fall asleep under these conditions. You can try to mark off an area that is just for sleeping with a curtain or screen. Covering up televisions and other materials at bedtime can also show everyone that it is time for bed.

Making Changes to the Sleep Environment

We talked about considering the following features of your child's sleep environment when we were evaluating her sleep in Chapter 4:

- temperature
- textures
- scents
- sounds
- light
- objects

We now want to think about what changes you can make so that these features help to promote sleep.

Temperature: We all tend to sleep better in cooler rather than warmer rooms. Think about your own child's preferences. Remember, if you use something like a fan, an air filter, or a heater that makes noise, it should remain on all night. You need to keep the machine on all night so that the sound remains consistent. If there is a change in sound after your child falls asleep, she will be more likely to wake up during the night.

Textures: Some children are sensitive to certain fabrics and prefer specific types of pajamas and bedding. Try to provide your child with what she prefers, if you can. Use fabrics that are comfortable for her and consider whether she might like looser- or tighter-fitting pajamas. If your child is sensitive to tags in her clothing, be sure to remove them from her pajamas. If she still wears diapers or pull-ups to bed, consider how comfortable they are. Some children wake up if their diaper or pull-up leaks, so it helps to make sure your child has a diaper or pull-up that fits well. It sometimes helps to have your child wear extra padding or plastic training pants for additional protection at night.

Some children like extra weight on their bodies at bedtime. Children who enjoy deep pressure and big hugs often respond well to using several blankets instead of just one. A weighted blanket may also be a good option. One way to determine whether a weighted blanket might work is to try using several blankets. Adding one or two blankets at a time makes it easier to tell if your child likes the extra weight.

Cotton or cloth sleeping bags are another good option for adding weight and comfort. Nylon sleeping bags tend to be too slippery. Some children even enjoy being squeezed into a sleeping bag with extra pillows inside the sleeping bag. We have also worked with children who enjoy sleeping in a tent. The closed-in feeling is often comforting to them. A sleeping bag or weighted blanket may also help children who are restless sleepers. If you do try any of these methods, please remember to think about any safety issues related to the materials in a weighted blanket or any ventilation issues related to the use of a sleeping bag or tent. You may also want to consult with your health care provider about the size and heaviness of a weighted blanket, as well as the type of filling that you use.

Scents: Some scents can be calming for children. Linking a specific scent to bedtime is another way to teach a child that it is time to go to bed. You can use soaps or spices in a small container to provide some relaxing scents for your child. You can also try filling a spray bottle with water and adding a few drops of scented oil. Make sure that these are kept out of your child's reach and in a safe place.

Sounds: Think about noises in the house. Some children with ASD are not sensitive to sound, but others are very aware of even small changes in the noise level. Playing music or using a noise machine may mask other sounds in the house. Remember that anything that makes noise needs to stay on all night. There are many products and apps that can be used for noise machines. Families can also make their own recordings of special songs or sounds and have them play on a tape loop all night. For children who do not respond well to ongoing noise and are sensitive to sounds, try blocking noise with extra padding around doors and windows.

Anthony slept well during the summer months but had trouble sleeping once the cold winter season began. His parents thought carefully about his room. They recalled that they used a fan in

Anthony's room in the summer. The fan made a comforting white noise that masked other sounds in the house. When the fan was turned off in the winter, he had trouble falling asleep. His family made a tape recording of the fan. They played this all night during the winter, and Anthony slept well.

Light: We want as little light as possible in a child's room while she is sleeping. Nightlights are fine for children who need them. Consider light from outside a child's room as well as the light that is in the room. Light coming in from a window or hallway can sometimes be very bright. Heavy curtains on the windows can make a big difference.

Some children are fearful of the dark and have gotten used to sleeping with the lights on. Children can learn to sleep with less light, although it can be a slow and gradual process. Consider using a dimmer switch or putting in light bulbs with lower and lower wattage over time.

Be sure to think about light from other sources, including televisions, computers, and electronic devices. If they are left on, they may produce light that will make it hard for your child to sleep. They also provide a tempting alternative to settling down and falling asleep! It would be best to remove these objects from your child's room. If that's not possible, consider covering them with a blanket at bedtime. You can set some electronic devices on timers so that they are automatically disabled at a specific time. This can help some children accept the idea that they can't play with these devices after a certain time. Teens may really resist putting their computers, phones, and games away for the night. Working together with your teen to set a realistic bedtime along with some limits about what happens once it is time to go to sleep is often effective.

Objects: Consider whether toys and other objects should be taken out of the bedroom or put away for the night. If your child is tempted to play with toys at bedtime, it might be best to remove them. Also think about what toys are in your child's bed. Some children need to put many treasured objects in bed with them before they fall asleep. As long as this does not interfere with sleep, it is not a problem. If it makes it hard for your child to fall asleep, consider limiting the number of objects she can take to bed. Sometimes it can be easier to make these changes little by little over time rather than all at once.

Frequently Asked Questions

Q: *What do I do if my child's bedtime routine has to change?*

A: It is OK to make changes from time to time. You might have to make changes when you first start your child's bedtime routine. An activity that you thought would be relaxing might be exciting instead. Make whatever changes you need to make. Once you have a good routine, it is best to try to stick to it for as long as you can. Once your child understands the bedtime routine, she might ask to make some changes. As long as the routine promotes good sleep, it will be good to involve her in the process. She might even want to help you make new images for her schedule!

If you have to make a change for just one night, that is OK, too. Try to make a visual aid to help your child make the change. This could be a picture of the new activity or an object used in the activity. If you are changing the order of your child's routine, make sure she knows about the new schedule. You could use a card or object that shows that there will be a change. For example, you could use a picture of a triangle to let your child know that something will be different. Put the triangle card in front of the new pictures or the new order of activities.

Q: *What is the best way to handle the change from standard time to daylight saving time and back again?*

A: Daylight saving time can be difficult for everyone! You can start to make slow changes to your child's sleep schedule about a week or so before the change. If you have established a regular bedtime routine for your child, it will be easier to help her deal with the time change. It will help to start a week or so before the actual time change occurs. Here's an example in which the clocks will move forward one hour for daylight saving time:

Let's say your child usually goes to bed at 8:00 p.m. and wakes up at 6:30 a.m. The time change will occur on a Sunday, so you will start changing your child's sleep and wake time earlier in the week. On Monday and Tuesday of that week, you will wake her up at 6:15 a.m. and put her to bed at 7:45 p.m. Other than changing the time, you will stick to your regular bedtime routine. On Wednesday and Thursday, you can wake her up at 6:00 a.m. and put her to bed at 7:30 p.m. On Friday and Saturday, you will wake her up at 5:45 a.m. and put her to bed at 7:15 p.m. Then on Sunday, you will wake her up at 7:00 a.m. (this is the new time) and have her go to bed at the new time of 8:00 p.m.

It will help if you set your clocks back on Saturday night so that everyone wakes up to the new time on Sunday morning. You might also consider moving dinner to a slightly earlier time each night as well. At the end of daylight saving time, you would reverse the process.

Q: *My daughter Ella likes to take a bath in the evening. She is calm in her bath until it is time to be done, but always becomes very upset when bath time is over. Should a bath be part of her bedtime routine?*

A: This could be a nice part of Ella's bedtime routine. The key will be to make sure bath time ends on a positive note. Make sure that Ella knows that she will get to do something fun when she gets out of her bath. Let her see her bedtime schedule. You can show her a picture or an object that tells her what she will do next. If she likes to read, you can show her one of her favorite books before you tell her it is time to finish her bath. You can use a timer to help her know it is time to be done. Teach her that when the timer goes off, she needs to get out of her bath. If these ideas don't work, you can move her bath earlier in the evening so that she has time to recover from the upset of ending this activity.

Q: *I have more than one child. My other children are interested in using a visual schedule, too! Is this OK, or should I keep it as a special activity for my child with ASD?*

A: It is great that your other children are interested in using a visual schedule! They may also benefit from developing a consistent bedtime routine, and they may help your child with ASD learn to use her schedule. Each child's bedtime routine can be individualized, and your children can each go through their own schedules at the right time for them. You can also enlist your children's help in making sure your child with ASD is engaging in calm and soothing activities before bed. You can help them know what types of activities are best, and even reward other children in the family for encouraging your child with ASD to participate in these activities.

References

1. W. J. Warzak, S. Evans, M. T. Floress, A. C. Gross, and S. Stoolman, "Caffeine Consumption in Young Children," *Journal of Pediatrics* 158, no. 3 (2011): 508–09.
2. K. Frank, K. Beck, and B. A. Malow. *Sleep Tool Kit for Children with Autism Spectrum Disorders.* Washington, DC: U.S. Department of Health and Human Services, Health Resources and Services Administration, Maternal and Child Health Research, 2011.

Books about Addressing Anxiety in Children

Chalfant, Anne M. *Managing Anxiety in People with Autism: A Treatment Guide for Parents, Teachers, and Mental Health Professionals.* Bethesda, MD: Woodbine House, 2011.

Chansky, Tamara E. *Freeing Your Child from Anxiety: Powerful, Practical Solutions to Overcome Your Child's Fears, Worries, and Phobias.* New York: Broadway Books, 2004.

Manassis, Katharina. *Keys to Parenting Your Anxious Child.* 2nd ed. Hauppauge, NY: Barron's Educational Series, 2008.

Books about Relaxation Techniques for Children

Cautela, Joseph R., and Groden, June. *Relaxation: A Comprehensive Manual for Adults, Children, and Children with Special Needs.* Champaign, IL: Research Press Company, 1978.

Shapiro, Lawrence E., and Sprague, Robin K. *The Relaxation and Stress Reduction Workbook for Kids: Help for Children to Cope with Stress, Anxiety & Transitions.* Oakland, CA: New Harbinger Publications, 2009.

Chapter 7

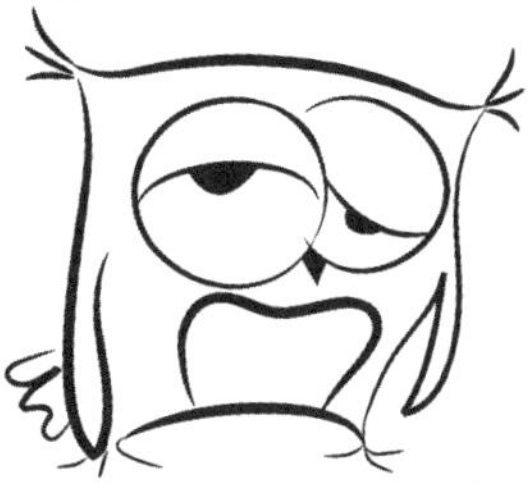

Falling Asleep and Staying Asleep

In the last chapter we discussed a number of different ways to get your child ready for bed. These include working on the elements of successful sleep, establishing a calming bedtime routine, and choosing the right bedtime—all of which should make going to sleep more pleasant and less stressful. For many children with ASD, these steps will lead to a good night's sleep. Other children need more support to fall asleep.

Why Does My Child Resist Going to Bed?

Some children with an ASD are able to easily fall asleep on their own in their own beds. Other children struggle to learn this skill, and their families try many different ways to get their children to go to sleep any way that they can. Some families allow their children to fall asleep on the couch or in their bed while watching television. Some children need motion to fall asleep and will fall asleep while their parents rock them or while they are sitting in a swing. Other children cannot fall asleep unless they are riding in the car, and their parents drive them around during the night. Many children need to fall asleep with a parent or other family member next to them.

While these habits allow a child to fall asleep, they are often very hard on families and may not promote sleep throughout the night. This is because we need whatever helped us fall asleep to be there to help us get back to sleep when we wake up at night. This is called a ***sleep onset association.***

We understand why mothers and fathers have used these strategies. They are loving parents who have done whatever it takes to help their children fall asleep. Often, they would like to make changes but don't know how. As parents learn about the importance of sleep associations and the need for their children to fall asleep on their own, they can work on other ways to promote sleep. With time and patience, they can teach their children new ways to fall asleep.

If your child has developed some sleep onset associations that you are ready to change, the suggestions in Chapter 6 will help your child develop new habits that make getting into bed easier than it has been in the past. But your child may still resist falling asleep! This is because many sleep onset associations are hard to break. It will take your child time to adjust to new routines and to your new expectations. Please be assured, however, that your child can learn new habits and learn to fall asleep on his own.

The first step is to think about why your child doesn't want to go to bed. Chapter 6 (Getting Ready for Bed) explains what to do if your child isn't sleepy at bedtime. These strategies will help all children with ASD sleep better, but those who are fearful may need some additional support.

How Can Your Child Learn to Sleep on His Own?

If you want your child to learn to sleep on his own, you need to give him the chance to learn this skill. This means giving him time alone in his bed to figure out how to do this. He'll need to spend time trying different ways to settle himself and get comfortable. The good news is that this doesn't take very long. Once your child has discovered a way to fall asleep on his own, he will always have this ability. You are giving him a lifelong gift.

There are three main ways to teach your child to fall asleep on his own:

- Crying It Out
- Checking In
- The Rocking Chair Method

Crying It Out

This is a traditional method, and it is also called ***extinction.*** We talked about extinction in Chapter 3. Once you say goodnight to your child, you do *not* go back in to talk with him or be with him, no matter what he does.

Although this method may work for very young children, there are several reasons we don't recommend this plan for parents of children with autism spectrum disorders. First, parents often find this method difficult to use. It is hard for parents to leave their child when they know that he is upset and fearful, and children with ASD often have significant difficulties with anxiety. Second, even if parents are willing to try this method, they often end up going into their child's room to provide comfort and support. If this happens, the method can backfire and work against the child and family! This is because the child learns that he just needs to be upset for some period of time before his parents will come to him. The end result is that he is still falling asleep with his parents' help. He has now also learned that some negative behaviors can work to help him get what he wants or needs. Thus, while "crying it out" works with some children, we do not recommend it for children with ASD.

Checking In

The "checking in" method is also called ***modified extinction.*** When you use this method, you say goodnight and leave the room (just as in the "crying it out" method). If your child is upset, you wait just a few minutes and then go back in. You are comforting, but your contact with him is "brief and boring." You try to keep the time you are with your child to under a minute. You say something like, "I love you. It's time to go to sleep. Goodnight." Using this method, you can go back into your child's room as often as needed. Over time, you lengthen the time between visits. This method may work for children with ASD, but it can be upsetting for children who are anxious.

The Rocking Chair Method (Fading Parental Presence)

We like this method best. We call it the "rocking chair" method, and learned it from Dr. Susan McGrew. Parents can sit in any type of chair when they try this approach. Some parents sleep on a mattress in their child's room instead of sitting in a chair. They are just too tired to sit in a chair!

You begin by saying goodnight to your child, but you don't leave the room. You sit with your back to your child and limit all contact (once again, the key words are "brief and boring.") With this method, you don't talk to or touch your child while he is falling asleep. Each night you move your chair a little farther away from his bed and closer to the door. A good last step is to let your child see some part of you (a hand or a foot) while you are mostly out in the hallway. Once you have finished this step, you are all done. Some children will actively take part in this plan. They will measure how far their parents are sitting away from them. This method slowly builds a child's self-confidence and lets him realize that he can sleep on his own.

While it is easiest for parents to start the "rocking chair" method seated in a chair near their children's bed, some children need a slower approach. This may be especially true for children who have been sleeping in the same bed with a parent. In this instance, you may need to start by sitting on your child's bed and then move slowly away from his bed. Some children need something to cuddle if they aren't snuggling with their parents. A large stuffed toy, a body pillow, or comfort objects are good substitutes. It might help to think about what your child does when he cuddles with you. If he likes to stroke your arm, you might give him a soft blanket with a satin edge to rub. If he likes playing with your hair, he might prefer a doll or stuffed animal that has long hair or fur that he can twist. As we've discussed, some children also benefit from using weighted blankets or sleeping bags. Your child might enjoy decorating his own bedding.

When Should I Work on Teaching My Child to Sleep on His Own?

The best time to teach your child how to fall asleep on his own is usually after he has established some other sleep habits. You might start by looking at the ideas in Chapter 6. Think about what will promote good sleep for your child. Work on the timing of bedtime, as well as your child's daytime behavior, evening routines, and bedtime schedule. It will be easier for your child to learn to fall asleep by himself after you have addressed these factors. He will be calmer and more ready for sleep.

Begin at Bedtime

As discussed in Chapter 4, psychologist V. Mark Durand advises that to help children sleep through the night, we need to "begin at bedtime."[1] A child who can fall asleep on his own can go back to sleep on his own. As we explained in Chapter 1, we all cycle through different phases of sleep throughout the night. As we move from one phase to another, we may naturally arouse from our sleep. If we have practiced falling asleep on our own at the beginning of the night, we can fall back asleep during the night. But, if we fall asleep by using something (or someone) that won't be there as we cycle through the different sleep phases, we are likely to wake up and become alert. Helping your child learn to fall asleep on his own at the beginning of the night is the best way to help him stay asleep through the night.

This does not mean that your child cannot cuddle with you before he goes to sleep. The key is to make sure that your child is falling asleep without any physical contact with you. Some parents snuggle with their children until they see that they are getting drowsy. They then move away from their child's bed (while still staying close by) so that he can learn how to fall asleep on his own. You want to give your child the time he needs to settle and fall asleep on his own. That way, he can use these strategies throughout the night to stay asleep. Remember, if a child falls asleep with his parents, he will need them with him all night in order to remain asleep. You can gradually increase the time between cuddling and putting your child in his bed so that eventually you are putting him to bed when he is not drowsy. You can use this same strategy to help your child be less dependent on many different sleep associations. He can listen to music, have a drink from a bottle, or be rocked back and forth until he is just starting to nod off. Just be sure to put him to bed on his own before he actually falls asleep.

The Bedtime Pass

Using a "Bedtime Pass" may also lessen anxiety and promote your child's ability to sleep on his own. This method was developed by Patrick Friman.[2] It appeals to the visual strengths of children with ASD and also their sense of control.

The bedtime pass is a small card that has a picture on one side and the words "bedtime pass" on the back. The size of the card can vary, but it is usually the size of a postcard or even smaller. See Figure 7.1 for a picture of a bedtime pass.A child receives a pass when he first goes to bed in the evening. If he has his pass when he wakes up in the morning, he can trade it in for a small prize. If he needs to check in with his parents, he needs to give up his pass. Bedtime passes can be used for a brief visit with a parent; these might include getting a drink of water, getting one last hug, or getting one last bedtime kiss. Even when a child gives his mother or father his bedtime pass, the parent keeps all contact brief and boring. A child cannot use his bedtime pass to sleep in his parent's bed! Once a child uses his pass, parents must ignore other attempts he makes to get their attention. If he comes out of his room, they guide him back to his bed with as little interaction as possible. Some children may need to start with more than one pass if they are in the habit of calling for their parents many times throughout the night.

It can be fun to decide on pictures for the bedtime pass! Parents and children may choose a picture that shows a child's special interest, or it can just be a picture that does not have any special meaning. Some children love the picture on their bedtime pass so much that they have slept with it under their pillows.

Your child might enjoy making a pass with you. You can easily make a bedtime pass by finding a picture in a magazine or on a website. You can also illustrate your own pass or have your child make his own drawing. You can then cover it with contact paper or laminate to protect it from wear and tear.

Figure 7.1—Bedtime Pass

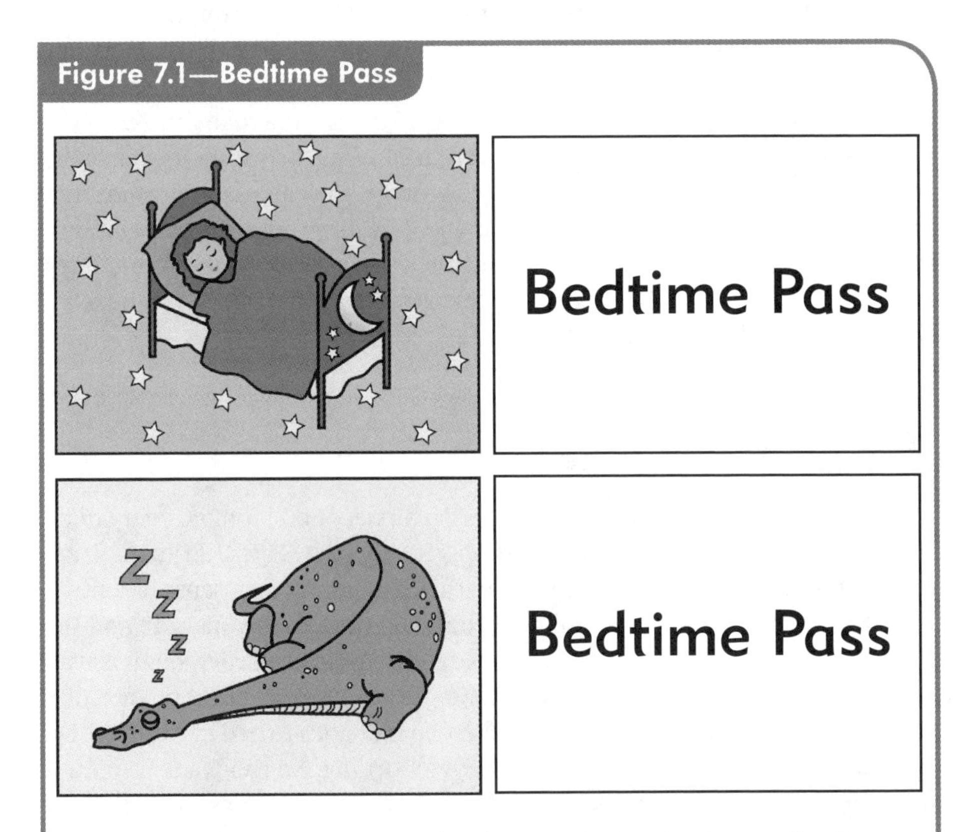

This sample bedtime pass and other examples in Appendix G were developed by Vanderbilt Kennedy Center's Treatment and Research Institute for Autism Spectrum Disorders (kc.vanderbilt.edu/triad) and was based on the work of Dr. Patrick Friman. They may also be found in the free *Sleep Booklet-Parent Booklet and Quick Tips* of the Autism Treatment Network/ Autism Intervention Research Network on Physical Health (ATN/AIR-P)

(http://www.autismspeaks.org/science/resources-programs/autism-treatment-network/tools-you-can-use/sleep-tool-kit).[3]

Using a bedtime pass gives some children the confidence they need to stay in bed without being with their parents. Knowing that they can use their pass to see their parents helps some children decide whether they really need to see mom or dad or whether they can wait until morning and receive a prize. Here is a story you can use to teach your child how to use a bedtime pass:

> *Mommy has given me a bedtime pass. The bedtime pass can help me stay in bed when it is time for sleep. I can use the bedtime pass to ask for a drink or to get out of bed. I keep my bedtime pass with me to use if I need to get up. If I use my bedtime pass to get up I have to give it to Mommy. If I use my bedtime pass to get a drink of water I have to give it to Mommy. If I keep my bedtime pass and stay in bed, I can get a treat in the morning when I wake up. I feel good when I can trade in my bedtime pass for a treat in the morning.*

You can find another story about bedtime passes and more examples of bedtime passes in the *Sleep Booklet-Parent Booklet and Quick Tips* available from the Autism Treatment Network/Autism Intervention Research Network on Physical Health (ATN/AIR-P) (http://www.autismspeaks.org/science/resources-programs/autism-treatment-network/tools-you-can-use/sleep-tool-kit). This resource and a variety of other tool kits are available free of charge from the ATN/AIR-P. They can be downloaded at http://www.autismspeaks.org/family-services/tool-kits.

You can use lots of different types of rewards when your child uses the pass successfully. You don't have to give him a big reward. It can be something small or it can be a chance to participate in a favorite activity. Some children respond well to earning stickers that can then be traded in for a larger reward. We discuss rewards more later in this chapter.

You can also use the bedtime pass to address night wakings. One of the most important things you can do to reduce night wakings is to work with your child to teach him to fall asleep on his own. If, for example, a child falls asleep by cuddling with one of his parents at the beginning of the night, he may awaken during the night when they are no longer in his bed and he cannot cuddle more to fall back asleep. If you use a bedtime pass to help with night wakings, make sure that you are helping your child develop sleep associations that allow him to fall asleep on his own at the beginning of the night. He will wake up less and will not need to see you as much if he is able to soothe himself and get back to sleep on his own.

How to Use the Bedtime Pass

Here are steps to take if you want to use the bedtime pass with your child:

1. Show a sample pass to your child and tell him how it works. (You and your child can make his own special pass together if you think he will enjoy this.)
2. Work with your child to choose some rewards he can get if he keeps his pass.
3. Give your child his pass at bedtime.
4. Remind him how it works.
5. If your child gets out of bed or asks to see you, give him a loving and short response and take his pass.
6. If your child gets out of bed once you have taken his pass, gently take him back to bed and keep your contact with him "brief and boring."
7. Give your child a reward in the morning if he has kept his pass all night.
8. Combine any prizes with lots of praise.

If your child does wake up during the night, respond quickly to any signs of distress but make sure your time with him is short. You still want to remember the "brief and boring" rule for all contacts during the night. You can certainly comfort your child, but do so with a quick "I love you; it's time to go back to sleep." While you will want to respond if your child is upset, be careful not to respond too quickly to ordinary arousals. These might include mild sleep talking or gentle tossing and turning. Sleeping in a room near your child or using an audio monitor will let you know when to ignore him and when to go to his room to see him. Remember to keep the lights down low if your child wakes up during the night.

At times, night wakings will get worse before they get better. Children may test the new plan to see how it really works. So, you might actually see more night wakings at first. Changes may not come instantly, but they will come. Consider your child's current sleep behavior and develop practical goals that reflect small and steady progress. If your child has been waking up several times a night, you can be encouraged if this decreases even a little after the testing phase has occurred. If you are using a bedtime pass, you might consider giving your child more than one pass to start with if he has been waking up several times a night. You could, for example, give him two passes and reward him if he still had one pass in the morning. This way he could achieve some success while slowly learning to stay in bed all night.

Other Visual Strategies

Some children with ASD benefit from the use of other visual strategies in addition to the bedtime pass. One strategy is to put a stop sign on the inside of your child's door at the start of the night and explain to him that he needs to stay in his room until you take the sign down in the morning. You can also use a light with a timer and set the timer to the morning time when it is OK for your child to get up from bed. Then you can let your child know that he needs to stay in his bed until the light turns on. Once again, we recommend rewarding your child in the morning for following this plan.

Transitioning Your Child to His Own Bed

The strategies we have been discussing will also work if your child has been sleeping in your bed and you want him to move to his own bed. You might start by working with your child to decorate his room so that he is excited about sleeping there. He might enjoy sheets or pictures that reflect his special interests.

Once he moves to his own bed, you may need to stay in his room while he gets used to sleeping there. You can sit near his bed and use the "rocking chair" method to gradually move back out of his room. Make sure that you help him develop good sleep associations that allow him to fall sleep on his own. You can also have your child gradually move out of your bed and into his own bed. Here are the steps to follow:

1. Begin by sleeping in your bed but with a body pillow or other bedding separating you and your child. The idea is to keep your child from needing to cuddle with you while he falls asleep.
2. Next have your child sleep in a separate bed (or in a sleeping bag) in your bedroom.
3. Over the course of several days, slowly move your child's bed away from your bed.
4. Let your child sleep in the hallway near your bedroom.
5. Move your child down the hallway toward his own bedroom little by little.
6. Move your child back into his own bedroom.

It is always essential to consider safety issues when your child awakens during the night. You might consider using audio or video monitors. You can also put a bell or other noise-making device on your child's door so you know if he leaves his room. Be sure to keep doors and cabinets locked and all dangerous objects safely out of reach. At times it may be helpful to consider using a zippered enclosure or safety bed that has been approved by your health care provider to help keep your child from wandering during the night.

Nightmares

Nightmares are a common part of childhood. They tend to happen in the later part of the night. When children wake from having nightmares, they are upset and may be able to talk about parts of their bad dreams. Children with minimal verbal skills may not be able to talk about their nightmares, but they will be wide awake and distressed.

Children tend to have bad dreams when they are upset or worried. The strategies described in Chapter 6 that promote a calm and relaxing bedtime may also reduce the number of nightmares that your child has. Using relaxation strategies can also make a difference.

What should you do if your child wakes up from a bad dream? We suggest comforting him a little and then having him go back to sleep. It is best to use a calm and supportive tone. Keep the conversation short and maintain your "brief and boring" stance. If your child sleeps in his own bed during the night, have him return to his bed. Don't change your child's nighttime routine because of nightmares. It can be tempting to let your child sleep with you or provide lots of extra attention after a bad dream, but this can often lead to new sleep habits that can be difficult to change.

You can decide whether you need to talk more about the bad dream the next day. Sometimes it isn't needed. If your child wakes up feeling fine, there is no reason to revisit what happened at night. At other times, your child may need an extra hug or a chance to talk about his feelings. If he has had a disturbing dream, you could ask him to draw a picture of what he remembers. This might be a good strategy for some children with limited language skills. It is still good to maintain a matter-of-fact attitude while talking about bad dreams during the day. Be sure to talk about nightmares well before bedtime.

Parasomnias

As you might recall from Chapter 5, parasomnias are different from nightmares. The main thing to remember about parasomnias is that your child is not actually awake. He may call out or cry loudly, and he may even walk around the house. He won't respond when you talk with him or try to comfort him, and he doesn't seem to be aware of your presence.

Parasomnias tend to occur earlier in the night (while nightmares occur in the latter part of the night), and your child will not remember these events. Night terrors are much more difficult for the people who are up than for the person who is asleep! Your child may be crying and screaming and seem quite distressed.

It is usually hard to comfort a child who is having a night terror, while it is easier to comfort someone who has had a bad dream. The best thing to do during these episodes is to make sure that your child is safe. Don't try to wake him up, but do try to guide him back to bed if this is needed. As we discussed in Chapter 5, parasomnias may be a sign of poor sleep throughout the night, so be sure to let your child's health care provider know about these behaviors.

Waking Up Early

Waking up very early in the morning is different from waking up during the night. Some children are ready for the day much earlier than the rest of their family is. They have slept through the night and are simply no longer tired. If your child used to sleep later in the morning and has just started waking up early, try to figure out whether anything has changed for him. Early morning awakenings may be associated with depression or anxiety. Think carefully about whether your child may be sad or upset about any recent or upcoming events. Sometimes early morning waking occurs if a child is anticipating transitions or big changes. Some examples include the beginning and end of the school year, exams, seasonal changes, problems with friends, or a new schedule. If you do identify something that might be stressful for your child, addressing the issue may help him sleep longer during the night.

If waking up early is just your child's natural sleep pattern, you have some choices about how to handle this:

- You can just accept this pattern and teach your child what to do when he wakes up early. Give him a box of materials that he can use during that early morning time.
- You can use a picture schedule or written list to help your child remember the activities he is permitted to do early in the morning. Use visual cues so that he knows when he can leave his bedroom and start his day.
- As suggested earlier, you can put a stop sign on his door when you say goodnight to him and then take it off in the morning when it is time for everyone to be up.

- You could also set a light or electronic device on a timer. When the light or device goes on, it is OK to get up for the day. You can also purchase special alarm clocks for children that produce a colored light in the morning.
- Consider using a story to help your child understand what you expect. See the example in the box below.
- You might also want to provide some rewards for your child when he stays in his room until an acceptable time.

William's Morning Plan

When I wake up in the morning I stay in my room until Mommy comes to say "Good Morning!" I can open my basket and play with my toys. I will play quietly because Mommy and Daddy need to sleep in the morning. When the stop sign is on my door, it means that I need to stay in my room. When the stop sign is gone, I can leave my room.

You can also try letting your child go to bed later at night. If your child falls asleep later, he will probably sleep longer in the morning. You can decide what hours you would most like your child to be asleep. This method works best with children who sleep all night without any interruptions. Here is an example:

Grace goes to sleep at 8:00 p.m. and wakes up at 4:00 a.m. each night. Her parents would like her to sleep later in the morning. They decide that they would like her to wake up at 5:30 a.m. at the earliest. Each night they make her bedtime a little later. They start by having her go to bed at 8:15 p.m. instead of 8:00 p.m. Grace falls asleep right away and sleeps until 4:15 a.m. After a few nights, her parents put Grace to bed at 8:30 p.m. She still falls asleep right away and now sleeps until 4:30 a.m. Her family continues to slowly change Grace's bedtime until she is falling asleep at 9:30 p.m. and waking up at 5:30 a.m.

Win Them Over!

How do you get your child to accept the changes that need to be made? Giving children small rewards for learning new sleep habits is an essential part of starting a new program. When your child wakes up in the morning, let him know that he has done a good job falling asleep on his own and provide him with a small prize. The rewards do not need to be big or costly. Your child might earn stickers or the chance to choose his favorite cereal at breakfast. It can also be fun to wrap up small prizes in colorful paper and have your child choose a surprise from a basket. If there is time in the morning, your child might earn time to play a preferred game or activity.

Small rewards often work wonders. Here are some different types:

Social	■ Play a board game ■ Cuddle ■ Talk on the phone ■ Play a chase game ■ Read a book together
Sensory	■ Back rubs ■ Smelling scents ■ Holding a warm blanket fresh from the dryer ■ Playing with water ■ Watching a fan turn round and round
Activities	■ Watching television ■ Watching a movie ■ Listening to music ■ Playing a computer game ■ Going outside
Objects	■ Food ■ Stickers ■ Cars ■ Blocks ■ Game cards

Once your child has successfully earned some rewards each morning, you can begin to fade out the daily rewards. Instead, you can set up a reward system that will allow him to earn some rewards over time. You might give him a sticker or a check mark on a special chart when he does what he needs to do at bedtime or during the night. When he has a certain number of stickers or checks, he can receive a prize from you.

When you are first teaching your child a new skill, it is best to give him a reward every morning. For example, the first time your child is able to keep his bedtime pass all night, be sure to give him a prize that morning. After he is able to keep his pass for several nights, you can move to a system where he needs to earn a certain number of stickers before he gets a prize. You might want to include your other children in this plan and give them prizes for sleeping well too. This might help motivate all your children to be good sleepers.

You can ask your child what he would like as prizes. You can purchase some inexpensive toys and wrap them up. Put the toys in a box and let your child choose a surprise when he wakes up in the morning.

Turn Things Around!

Think about some of your child's favorite evening activities. If these seem to make it harder for your child to fall asleep at night, try giving him time in the morning to do these activities. For example, if your child likes to watch an exciting television show right before bedtime, he can earn the chance to watch this show in the morning if he follows his bedtime routine.

It Is OK to Negotiate!

Some children are unwilling to go along with the changes that need to be made to improve their sleep. It is often very hard for children with ASD to give up watching television or playing a computer game before bed. Power struggles are always difficult, and it is best to avoid them before bed! Talk with your child and try to find the middle ground. There will be different solutions depending on what your child wants to do and what you want him to do. An example of how parents and children might meet halfway is shown in Figure 7.2.

If your child insists on participating in an activity that you are certain interferes with his sleep, or if he finds a way to do something that keeps him up at night, you may need to lock the object or activity away or disable it with a code or timer. You can also try having your child help you put the materials away and earn rewards for cooperation. Here's how Benjamin's parents handled this situation.

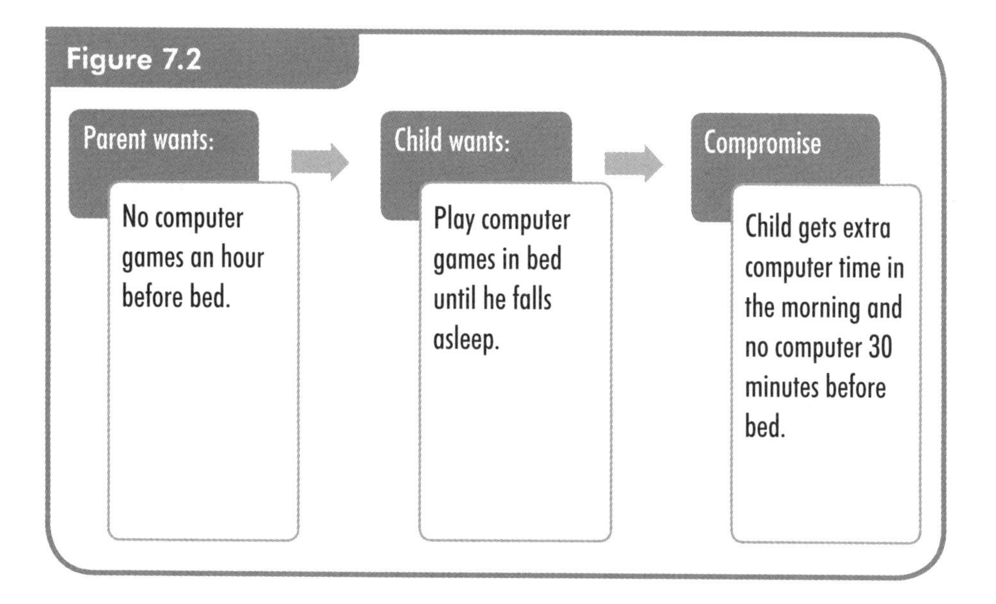

Twelve-year-old Benjamin liked to play on his smart phone long after he was supposed to go to sleep at 9:00 p.m. His parents decided that they needed to lock the phone away at the end of the evening. They knew that Benjamin would be upset about this new rule, so they decided to let him stay up until 10:00 p.m. He was allowed to play on his phone until 9:00 p.m., and then he had to give his phone to his parents. He would watch as they locked the phone away for the night. Benjamin earned a special bedtime snack for cooperating with this plan.

Frequently Asked Questions

Q: *My ten-year-old son insists on sleeping with his light on all night. He says he is afraid of the dark. He is able to fall asleep on his own, but it takes him a long time. I tried making the lights just a little dimmer, and he became very upset. What should I do?*

A: See if he will let you stay with him in his room with the lights turned off or dimmed. He may feel less anxious if you are there with him. He can then learn to fall asleep in the dark, and you can gradually decrease the amount of light in his room. Once he is able to fall asleep without any lights (or just a night light), you can gradually move out of his room using the "rocking chair" method.

Q: *My daughter Sophia is four years old. She drinks milk every night before bed and asks for milk many times during the night. I give her milk whenever she asks because I worry that she may be hungry. Is it OK to stop giving her milk at night?*

A: Unless they have a medical condition, children Sophia's age do not need to eat or drink during the night. In fact, eating and drinking during the night can make a child hungrier and make it even harder to sleep through the night. There are a few things you can do to make it easier to wean Sophia from her nightly milk-drinking habit:

1. Make sure Sophia is getting plenty of milk during the day. She may be less interested in drinking milk at night if she gets what she needs during the day. Check with your health care provider to make sure she does not drink too much milk in a twenty-four-hour period.
2. Offer Sophia milk as part of her bedtime routine.
3. Make sure that Sophia does not fall asleep while she is drinking.
4. Start to gradually decrease the amount of milk you give Sophia during the night. You can dilute her milk with water. You can also give her smaller and smaller amounts of milk.
5. Teach Sophia about using a bedtime pass. Write a story that tells her that she will get rewards for keeping her pass and not asking for a drink of milk.
6. Don't worry if Sophia asks for even more milk when you first start this program. Children (and adults!) often respond to limits by testing them and trying even harder to keep things the same.

Q: *My son Brandon has started waking up every night at 3:30 in the morning. He comes to my room and wants to talk and play. He doesn't have any trouble falling asleep at night. He falls asleep on his own at 7:30 p.m. every night. He also takes a nap every afternoon from 1:00 to 3:00. How can I help him sleep longer at night?*

A: Make sure that Brandon is not worried or depressed about something. Check to see if anything has changed that might be making him feel more stressed. Brandon is getting ten hours of sleep. This may be all he needs in a twenty-four-hour period. You could try making naptime shorter. You could also try putting him to bed later. He may then sleep later in the morning. You can also teach Brandon about using a bedtime pass. You can give him a box of toys that he can play with in the early morning. Consider putting his lights on a timer so that he will have a way of knowing when it is OK to leave his bedroom and see you.

Q: *I've always let my daughter sleep with me. I feel guilty that I want to change things, but now I want her to sleep on her own. She is six years old. Is it too late to teach her to do this?*

A: It is not too late! Please do not feel guilty. You are now ready to help your daughter learn a lifelong skill. She will be proud of herself, and you will get more sleep. It is often best to go slowly when teaching older children to sleep on their own. Consider using the "rocking chair" or "checking in" method. Review your daughter's daytime and evening habits to make sure she will be ready for sleep at bedtime. Make sure that you include some calm and relaxing activities in her bedtime routine. Let her help you decorate her room and make it a good place for sleep. You might want to put her to bed a little later so that she will be sleepy and more ready to fall asleep. Think about small rewards that you can give your daughter for learning new sleep habits. By taking the time to do this now, you are giving your daughter the gift of good sleep and the confidence to fall asleep on her own.

Q: *What is the best way to handle bedwetting?*

A: There are a few steps to take. First, it is very important to make sure your child doesn't have a medical condition that is related to his bed wetting. If this is a new problem, and there isn't a medical explanation, think about whether your child is anxious or upset about something. It is also important to consider your child's age. Many children under the age of six still wet their beds. If your child is older and has never been able to stay dry at night, there are some simple things you can do to help. Be sure to limit the amount he drinks before bedtime and have him go to the bathroom right before bed. Stay calm and matter-of-fact if an accident does occur. If these ideas don't help, you can develop a more intensive behavioral program with the help of your health care provider or a behavioral therapist. Some of these programs include scheduled awakenings and the use of an alarm (sometimes referred to as a "bell and pad.") There is a lot to consider when putting a program like this into place, and it really helps to have the support and expertise of a trained professional.

Q: *We want to use the bedtime pass with our child, but we're not sure how this will work if he needs to go to the bathroom during the night.*

A: Try giving your child two bedtime passes. One will just be for going to the bathroom (you can even put a picture of a toilet on this pass) and the other pass can be used in exchange for brief contact with you. This would include the usual activities we have talked about, such as a hug, a kiss, or a quick "I love you." If your child needs you when he goes to the bathroom, be sure to keep your contact brief and boring. You might also make sure that you or your child does not need to turn on any bright lights in order to go to the bathroom. You can put night lights in the hallway leading to the bathroom and in the bathroom itself. If you can limit how much your child drinks before bed, this might also decrease the need for him to use the bathroom during the night.

References

1. V. M. Durand, *Sleep Better! A Guide to Improving Sleep for Children with Special Needs,* rev. ed. (Baltimore: Paul H. Brookes, 2013): 111-12.
2. P. C. Friman, K. E. Hoff, C. Schnoes, K. A. Freeman, D. W. Woods, and N. Blum, "The Bedtime Pass: An Approach to Bedtime Crying and Leaving the Room," *Archives of Pediatrics and Adolescent Medicine* 153, no. 10 (1999): 1027-29.
3. K. Frank, K. Beck, and B. A. Malow. (2011). *Sleep Tool Kit for Children with Autism Spectrum Disorders.* Washington, DC: U.S. Department of Health and Human Services, Health Resources and Services Administration, Maternal and Child Health Research, 2011.

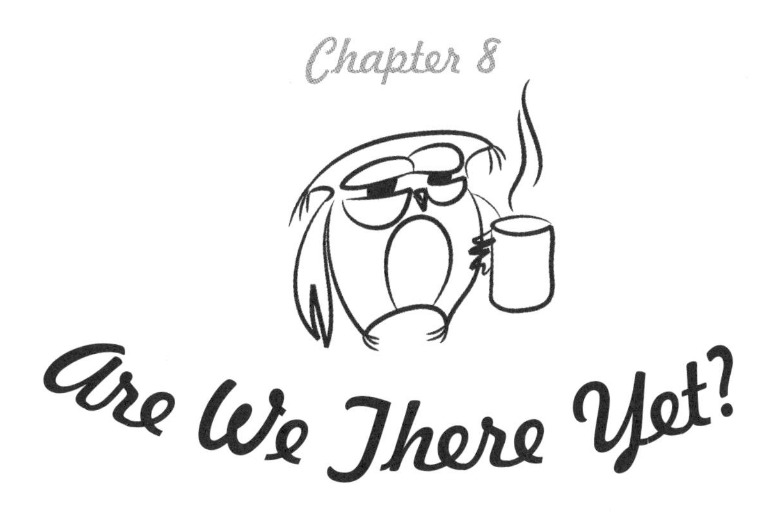

Chapter 8

Are We There Yet?

Let's review the steps you have taken to help improve your child's sleep:

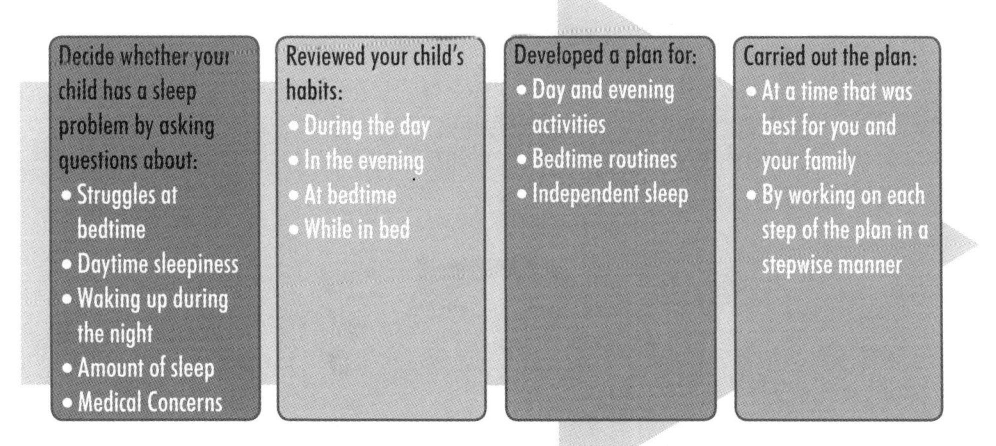

Once you have put a plan in place, you need to figure out how well it is working. There are a number of questions to answer:

- Is bedtime less of a struggle?
- Is your child falling asleep more quickly than before?
- Have nighttime awakenings decreased?
- Is your child learning to fall asleep on her own?
- Does she seem less tired during the day?
- Are there any remaining medical concerns?

Making changes to a program is part of the work!

Please don't feel discouraged if you need to adjust your sleep program. You may need to modify your plan based on how your child responds. This often needs to happen when you are working on changing routines and behaviors. It is an ongoing process of adapting your plan to fit your child's individual needs.

It takes time to make the changes described in earlier chapters and to see results. In general, you should expect to see some progress after just a few days. This doesn't mean that your child will instantly start falling asleep within twenty minutes of being put to bed. Progress may come in smaller steps, and any changes should be celebrated! First steps will usually involve your child struggling less with some of the changes to daytime and evening habits. Once some of these new strategies are in place, improvement in sleep should follow.

Don't be discouraged if your child becomes upset about some of the changes you are making. There is always something you can do to keep making progress. If you put a plan into action, you will learn something about what works and what doesn't work. You can then use this information to revise your plan.

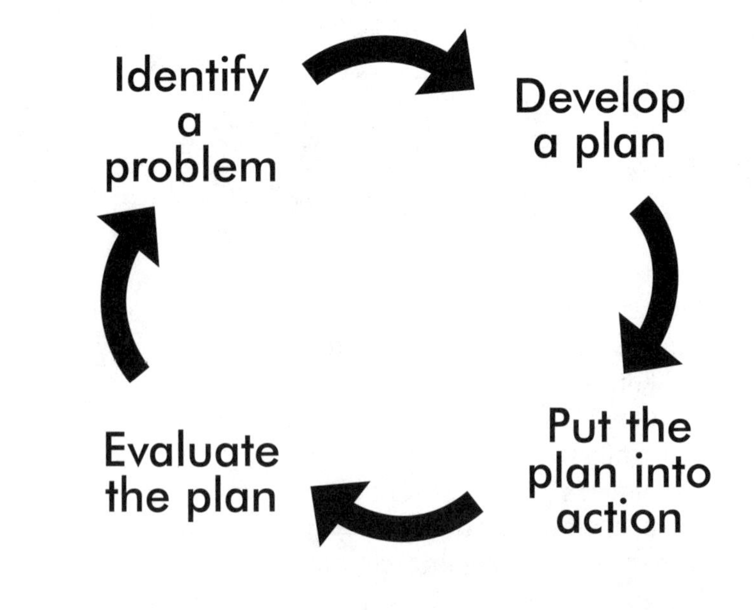

Troubleshooting When Your Plan Isn't Working

Sometimes you will know right away if a plan is working. Other times it helps to keep some notes about what strategies you are trying and how they are working. You can use the sleep record form that we have included in Appendix H to help you keep track of information. A copy of the form may also be downloaded or printed out from www.woodbinehouse.com/SolvingSleepProblems.asp.Using this form is one way to keep track of what is working and what is not working for your child. You can also just jot down some ideas, if that is easier.

Here are some questions to ask if your program is not turning out the way you would like:

- Are things moving at a good pace for your child?
- Is your child able to adjust to all the changes you have put into place?
- Did you prepare your child for the changes you have put into place?
- Have you covered all the ingredients of good sleep?
- Have medical reasons for poor sleep been considered?

Let's look at each of the questions above and discuss ways to alter your program as needed.

Are Things Moving at a Good Pace for Your Child?

Ideally, you have put a plan in place that makes it easy to succeed. You have started at a place where your child will be comfortable, and you have added changes slowly. You will know that you are moving too quickly if your child becomes distressed at the changes you are making. If this happens, usually all you need to do is step back and slow things down.

Here's an example of how this might work:

Ava liked to sleep with a bright light on in her bedroom closet. She took a long time to fall asleep at night, and her father decided that she would fall asleep more quickly if the light in her closet was less bright. First, he switched her 100-watt bulb for a 10-watt bulb, but Ava was very upset by this change. Her father realized that this was too abrupt a change for Ava; he installed a dimmer switch in her closet and let her sleep with the full 100-watt bulb for a few days. He then gradually started dimming the light so that the change was barely noticeable. By the end of two weeks, Ava was able to fall asleep comfortably when the light was on a low setting.

Is Your Child Able to Adjust to All the Changes You Have Put into Place?

We have presented many strategies that may make your child's sleep better. Some children can handle all of the changes at once, while others need to have each change added in a step-by-step manner. Children with ASD are often resistant to dealing with a lot of changes at the same time. If this is the case with your child, you can wait before making some of the changes. You can also give your child a choice about the changes in her routine.

Did You Prepare Your Child for the Changes You Put into Place?

Every child is different in terms of how much preparation she needs in order to accept change. Many children with ASD become anxious when faced with new routines, and visual aids may help them understand and accept change. If your child is resisting a new routine, it may be because she doesn't understand what she needs to do. Providing visual cues, physical structure, and opportunities for practice can make a big difference!

Jacob's parents were eager to have him use a visual schedule. They had heard about visual schedules, but had never used them before. When they first tried using a schedule with Jacob before bed, he became frustrated and confused. They reread how to teach children to use a visual schedule and decided that they had included too many activities. They simplified Jacob's schedule so it only included a few tasks. They also had him practice using a visual schedule during the day. They made some cards to show him what would happen after school, and he used his schedule to move from one fun activity to the next.

Once Jacob knew how to use a schedule, his parents tried it again at bedtime. This time, Jacob responded positively, and he was able to use his schedule each night before bed.

Have You Covered All the Ingredients of Good Sleep?

What if your child has accepted all of the changes that you've made, but she is still struggling with sleep? The first step is to go back through the ingredients of good sleep covered in Chapter 4 and make sure that you've covered all of the basics. For example, you may find that you need to work more on limiting lights at bedtime or you might need to double-check to see if your child is playing on her bed during the day. One way to keep track of what is working is to do some homework and keep a daily log of what is happening during the day, evening, and night. Using the sleep record form in Appendix H (and on the website) is one way to keep track of what is working and what is not working for your child.

Have Medical Reasons for Poor Sleep Been Considered?

You've put all the ideas we've discussed into place. You've reviewed and tweaked your plan. But your child is still not sleeping well. It may be time to go back to your health care provider and discuss any possible medical reasons for her sleep difficulties. Check for medication-related disruptions to sleep as well. If your child sees different specialists and perhaps gets medications from more than one provider, it is important that at least one of your providers be aware of all the medications, in case there are drug interactions.

We Were There...What Happened?

There could be a number of reasons why a child who has been sleeping well starts to have problems once again. Here are some possible reasons your child could start struggling with sleep again:

Changes in routine:

- A move to a new home
- Transitioning to a new classroom
- A change in friendship
- Starting a new club or sport
- A big test or assignment
- Family stressors such as illness, conflicts among family members, or changes in a parent's job
- Being teased or bullied at school (if you think this might be the case, talk with your child's teacher—some children have trouble telling their parents that they are having social difficulties)

Bodily changes:

- The onset of puberty
- An illness
- New medications
- Dental issues (such as getting braces or new molars)
- Allergies

- Reactions to the change in seasons
- Sensitivity to new cleaning products at home or school

What steps can you take?

Talk to your health care provider about any medical concerns.

- Confer with your child's school to identify and address any social or academic difficulties.
- Think about ways to help your child deal with new situations.
- Try to maintain consistent schedules and expectations during this period of change.
- Consult with a behavioral therapist or sleep specialist.

If your child has been sleeping well and suddenly starts having problems, don't despair! You and your child have developed the skills you need to help her sleep well. You just need to determine the reason for the change in her sleep and then help her reestablish good sleep habits.

At times it may be helpful to meet with someone who has training in behavioral intervention, autism spectrum disorders, and sleep difficulties. It can often be beneficial to get some additional advice and suggestions and to meet with someone who can provide a fresh perspective on your child's sleep difficulties.

Chapter 9

Sleeping Away from Home

It is fun and educational for children to go new places and see new things. We want to provide these types of opportunities for our children with ASD, and don't want sleep difficulties to interfere with their enjoyment. Many children with autism spectrum disorders have difficulty sleeping in new places, however. If your child develops good sleep habits at home, it may help him be able to sleep in a variety of situations, including:

- vacations
- sleep-away camp
- class trips
- sleepovers
- camping trips

Changes That Can Disrupt Sleep

Many factors can make it harder to sleep in a new place, including:

- new activities during the day
- changes in evening patterns
- altered bedtime routines
- different sleeping plans

We can identify strategies for success to improve your child's ability to sleep away from home by looking at each of these factors.

New Things to Do during the Day

Oftentimes, sleeping in a new place follows a day of novel events. While these new activities can be fun and exciting, they may cause a child with an autism spectrum disorder to experience some anxiety or uncomfortable feelings. Some children may become stressed by activities that are meant to be fun.

Changes in daily routines can disrupt sleep, but using visual schedules and writing individualized stories for your child in advance of the trip can make a positive difference. (See Chapter 6 for information about writing stories to help prepare your child for changes.) Also check to see if there are any online videos of the places that your child will visit. Consider whether you can give your child a break during the day to engage in some familiar and comforting activities.

Changes in Evening Activities

You have worked hard to develop an evening routine that incorporates calm and relaxing events as bedtime approaches. When your child is away from home, it is harder to provide the structure that will allow him to unwind. If possible, give your child a chance to have some downtime at the end of the day. Just like at home, turn the lights down low and encourage him to participate in his regular evening routines. Delaying bedtime so that your child has time to relax may help him fall asleep. This is, of course, harder to do when your child is not with you during the evening and at bedtime.

Disrupted Bedtime Routines

It is often difficult to follow a well-established bedtime routine in a new location. When your child can't follow his usual routine, he may feel anxious and have more trouble falling asleep. Whenever possible, think ahead to identify what parts of your child's bedtime routine will change, and try to keep the routine as consistent as possible. Using the same visual schedule you use at home will help. Use as many of the actual objects that are part of his bedtime routine as you can. For instance, make sure he has the same toothbrush, if this is part of his bedtime routine. This will be comforting to your child and help prepare him physically for sleep.

Different Sleeping Habits

Your child has gotten used to sleeping with his pillow, blanket, and other bedding at home. He may use a body pillow or a sleeping bag to help him fall asleep. Without these objects, he may have a lot of trouble falling asleep. Think about which articles he most needs at night and try to arrange for him to have them when he is sleeping away from home. Some examples might include his pillow case, nightlight, or noise machine.

Supports and Strategies to Make Sleeping Away from Home Easier

Some of the techniques that you use to help your child sleep better at home will also help him sleep in a new setting:

- stories that you write to help prepare him for new experiences
- videos
- photographs
- visual schedules
- practice
- rewards
- comfort objects

Let's see how we can use each of these techniques to help Sam sleep better during a trip to visit family in another state.

Sam's mother starts by writing a story about the trip:

I am taking a vacation. I am going to visit Uncle John, Aunt Rachel, and my cousins Jeremy and Kathy. I am going to fly on an airplane with Mommy and Daddy. We will play games and visit fun places during the day. At night we will have dinner and then have quiet time just like we do when we are home. Then it will be time for bed.

I am going to sleep in a hotel with Mommy and Daddy. I will sleep in my own bed. Mommy and Daddy will sleep in another bed that is near my bed. We will all sleep in the same room. When it is time for bed I will use my schedule to help me get ready. When I go into bed I will be quiet and try to fall asleep. I will cuddle with my bear while I am in bed. If I stay in my bed and sleep all night, I will get a prize in the morning. I am excited about going on a trip.

Sam's mother goes to the website of the hotel where they are planning to stay. She downloads videos and pictures to show Sam. She adds some of these pictures to the story she wrote for Sam and puts others in a book that includes pictures of other places they will visit while on vacation. While researching the hotel, she finds out whether she can request a quiet room that is far away from the elevator.

In addition to bringing Sam's regular bedtime schedule, his mother has made a new visual schedule that shows what Sam will do each day during their trip. She makes sure the schedule has a picture that represents quiet time before bed. Sam knows that when quiet time is over, he will use his bedtime schedule. His mother used some family photos as well as some that she found on the Internet and in magazines to complete Sam's schedule. Here is Sam's vacation schedule:

- Wake up.
- Get dressed.
- Eat breakfast.
- Visit Uncle John, Aunt Rachel, Jeremy, and Kathy.
- Eat lunch.
- Go to the zoo (afternoon activities will change each day).
- Eat dinner.
- Go back to the hotel.
- Quiet time.

Sam is used to sleeping in his own bed, so his mother is not sure how he will react to sharing a hotel room with his parents. She and Sam role play what it will be like to sleep in the same room. During the day she lies down in one bed while Sam lies down with his stuffed bear in another bed in the same room. She tells Sam that if he can lie quietly for five minutes, he will get a small prize. She then increases the time she asks Sam to do this until he is lying quietly for twenty minutes (which is about how long he usually takes to fall asleep).

Sam and his mother worked together to find some small prizes that he can earn for trying to fall asleep. She will bring these and his stuffed bear when they travel.

On the last day of their trip, his mother reads a new story to Sam. This story describes how he will sleep in his own room once he returns home.

The strategies described above will also work for other situations in which your child will sleep away from home. Please remember that many people have more trouble sleeping in a new location. Do what you can to help your child, but don't be too concerned if his sleep is disrupted. Once you return home, you will be able to help him return to the calming sleep routines that you have established.

Frequently Asked Questions

Q: *My daughter is going to sleep-away camp for the first time. What I can I do to help prepare her?*

A: Many of the strategies that Sam's mother used (see above) will be helpful for your daughter. Find out as much as you can about the camp schedule and how children sleep at the camp. Try to obtain videos and pictures so that you can help familiarize your daughter with the routine. Write a story about daytime, evening, and bedtime activities at camp. Find out in advance if you can make any special preparations to make her stay a success. Ask if she can use a visual schedule or bring any comfort objects with her. Try to role-play and practice camp routines, if possible. It may help to write a letter to the camp director letting him or her know about what might be most helpful for your daughter. Here is a sample letter:

Dear ________________________:

We are very excited that Olivia will be attending your camp. She loves nature and hiking. She is on the swim team at school and is looking forward to time on the lake. She is a good artist and often works on her own craft projects. We think your camp will be a wonderful experience for her!

As you know, Olivia has an autism spectrum disorder (ASD). She has had some sleep difficulties in the past but now has a good evening and bedtime routine that helps her sleep well through the night. We thought it would be helpful for you to know about her sleep habits. Olivia will probably sleep best if she can have some quiet time for about fifteen minutes before "lights out" time. She finds that reading is very relaxing for her. We are also hopeful that Olivia can use her bedtime visual schedule to guide her through her bedtime routine. She uses this schedule on her own, and it consists of typical bedtime tasks such as teeth brushing and putting on pajamas.

Finally, Olivia has a special pillow that she sleeps with. We are asking that she be able to use this pillow while she is at camp. Please let us know if these arrangements are acceptable. Thank you for your time and help.

Sincerely,
Olivia's parents

Q: *My son Jake really wants to have a sleepover with his best friend Antonio. Jake has a very strict bedtime routine, and I'm worried that a sleepover will really disrupt his sleep. What can I do?*

A: It may help to have Jake's first sleepover at your house instead of at Antonio's house. It will be easier for Jake to stick to his regular bedtime routine at your house, and you can see how Jake and Antonio interact at night. You can write a story about sleepovers and rehearse this with Jake. You can also practice some bedtime scenarios with him. After the sleepover at your house, you will have more information that you can use to help prepare Jake for a sleepover at Antonio's. You can share information with Antonio's mother to help the sleepover go smoothly. If Jake uses a picture schedule or needs some quiet time, you can talk with her about whether she would be comfortable helping him with this. You can also plan the sleepovers for days when it will be a little easier for Jake to get back on schedule after his fun night.

Q: *How should I handle a class trip that includes an overnight stay?*

A: Talk with your child's teacher about the best way to handle this. Find out what the sleeping arrangements will be and how children will be grouped together. Decide whether it would be best for your child to sleep in a room with an adult. See if your child can be paired with accepting peers who will be good role models. Discuss evening and bedtime routines and how these will work for your child. Once you have this information, rehearse different scenarios (through stories, role modeling, and practice) with your child. Also, remember that most children sleep less on school trips even when adults have the best intentions!

Q: *Our daughter, Chloe, is going to spend the week with her grandparents while we are on an adults-only vacation. Everyone is excited about this, but I have some concerns about Chloe's sleep schedule. My parents like to watch television late at night, and I do not want them to have to change what they do to relax in the evening. Chloe is a light sleeper, and she loves to watch television! How can I help Chloe sleep well while she is away?*

A: You can try using a noise machine to mask the sound. You might also talk with your parents about some small compromises that might help. Perhaps they can watch television with the door closed so that the noise is muted. They might also be able to use headphones so that only they can hear the sound. Finally, your parents could try putting Chloe in a bedroom that is far away from the television set.

Q: *What is the best way to handle bedtime when a babysitter will be putting our son to bed?*

A: Visual schedules help everyone stick to the same bedtime routine. Make sure your son's babysitter knows about your son's visual schedule and how to use it. You might want to have the babysitter come over one night when you are home and practice the bedtime routine with your son while you are present. Then, your son and his sitter will be able to go through the routine when you are away. If your child does not use a visual schedule, but has a consistent sensory routine that helps him transition to bedtime, you can practice that with your sitter as well.

Q: *My daughter is going to start spending weekends with my ex-husband. How can I help her maintain her good sleep habits?*

A: Talk with your ex-husband about your daughter's sleep routine and try to keep things at bedtime as consistent as possible between both homes. It would be best if you could agree on the same bedtime and wake time.

Appendix A
Sleep Surveys & Questionnaires

This appendix reviews some of the surveys and questionnaires that are commonly used to evaluate children's sleep habits and difficulties. We have also provided references for these surveys for readers who are interested in learning more about the different sleep surveys and how they help identify sleep problems in children and teens. You can use these surveys to help you decide if your child needs help with her sleep. You might also want to complete a survey and go over the answers with your child's health care provider to see if you need to address any medical issues about your child's sleep.

Surveys That Look at How Children Get to Sleep and Stay Asleep

- ***Adolescent Sleep Wake Scale.*** (LeBourgeois et al., 2005). This is a self-report measure for adolescents ages 12 to 18 with questions about going to bed, falling asleep, awakening, remaining asleep, and wakefulness.

  LeBourgeois, M. K., Giannotti, F., Cortesi, F., Wolfson, A. R., and Harsh, J. "The Relationship between Reported Sleep Quality and Sleep Hygiene in Italian and American Adolescents." *Pediatrics* 115, no. 1 (2005): 257–59.

- ***Children's Sleep Wake Scale.*** (LeBourgeois et al., 2001). This is a parent-report measure for parents of children ages 2 to 8 years that asks about going to bed, falling asleep, awakening, remaining asleep, and wakefulness.

  LeBourgeois, M.K., and Harsh, J. R. "A New Research Measure for Children's Sleep." *SLEEP 24 (2001):* A213–A214.

Surveys That Look at Daytime Sleepiness

- ***Cleveland Adolescent Sleepiness Questionnaire.*** (Spilsbury et al., 2007). This is a self-report measure of daytime sleepiness and alertness for children and adolescents ages 11 to 17.

Spilsbury, J. C., Drotar, D., Rose, C. L., Redline, S. "The Cleveland Adolescent Sleepiness Questionnaire: A New Measure to Assess Excessive Daytime Sleepiness in Adolescents." *Journal of Clinical Sleep Medicine* 3, no. 6 (2007): 603–12.

- ***Epworth Sleepiness Scale-Revised for Children.*** (Melendres et al., 2004; Moore et al., 2009). Child and parent report of daytime sleepiness for individuals ages 2 to 18.

  Melendres, M. C., Lutz, J. M., Rubin, E. D., Marcus, C. L. (2004). "Daytime Sleepiness and Hyperactivity in Children with Suspected Sleep-Disordered Breathing." *Pediatrics* 114, no.3 (2004): 768–75.

  Moore, M., Kirchner, H. L., Drotar, D., Johnson, N., Rosen, C., Ancoli-Israel, S., and Redline, S. "Relationships among Sleepiness, Sleep Time, and Psychological Functioning in Adolescents." *Journal of Pediatric Psychology* 34, no.10 (2009): 1175-83.

- ***Pediatric Daytime Sleepiness Scale.*** (Drake et al., 2003). This is a self-report measure of daytime sleepiness for children and adolescents ages 11 to 15. It may also be used with children as young as 5 years of age.

  Drake, C., Nickel, C., Burduvali, E., Roth, T., Jefferson, C., and Pietro, B. "The Pediatric Daytime Sleepiness Scale (PDSS): Sleep Habits and School Outcomes in Middle-School Children." *Sleep* 26, no. 4 (2003): 455–58.

- ***Teacher's Daytime Sleepiness Questionnaire.*** (Owens et al., 2000). This questionnaire asks teachers to report on daytime sleepiness of students ages 4 to 10 years of age.

  Owens, J. A., Spirito, A., McGuinn, M., and Nobile, C. "Sleep Habits and Sleep Disturbance in Elementary School-Aged Children. *Journal of Developmental and Behavioral Pediatrics* 21, no. 1 (2000): 27–36.

Surveys That Look at Sleep Habits

- ***Bedtime Routines Questionnaire.*** (Henderson & Jordan, 2010). A parent-report measure for parents of children ages 2 to 8 years of age.

  Henderson J., and Jordan, S. S. "Development and Preliminary Evaluation of the Bedtime Routines Questionnaire." *Journal of Psychopathology and Behavioral Assessment* 32 (2010): 271–80.

- ***Children's Sleep Hygiene Scale.*** (LeBorgeois & Harsh, 2001; Harsh et al., 2002). Parents of children ages 2 to 8 complete this questionnaire about their children's bedtime routines.

    LeBourgeois, M. K., and Harsh, J. R."A New Research Measure for Children's Sleep." *Sleep* 24 (2001): A360.

    Harsh, J. R., Easley, A., and LeBourgeois, M. K. "A Measure of Children's Sleep Hygiene." *Sleep* 25 (2002): A316.

- ***Family Inventory of Sleep Habits.*** (Malow et al., 2009). This questionnaire is specifically designed for parents of children with autism spectrum disorders ages 3 to 10. It is the only sleep measure geared toward children with autism spectrum disorders.

    Malow, B. A., Crowe, C., Henderson, L., McGrew, S. G., Wang, L., Song, Y., and Stone, W. L. "A Sleep Habits Questionnaire for Children with Autism Spectrum Disorders." *Journal of Child Neurology* 24, no. 1 (2009): 19–24.

Surveys That Look at Different Aspects of Sleep

- ***BEARS.*** (Owens & Dalzell, 2005). This is a pediatric screening questionnaire that asks adolescents or parents of younger children to answer five questions about sleep, including about the following: bedtime problems, excessive daytime sleepiness, awakenings during the night, regularity and duration of sleep, and snoring (see Appendix B for a full list of these questions).

    Owens, J. A., and Dalzell, V. "Use of the 'BEARS' Sleep Screening Tool in a Pediatric Residents' Continuity Clinic: A Pilot Study." *Sleep Medicine* 6 (2005): 63–69.

- ***Children's Sleep Habits Questionnaire.*** (Owens et al., 2000). This measure asks parents of children ages 2 to 10 to report on a number of different aspects of their sleep, including possible medical concerns. The questionnaire has also been validated with children with autism spectrum disorders ages 2 ½ to 5 years of age (Goodlin-Jones et al., 2008).

    Owens, J. A., Spirito, A., and McGuinn, M. "The Children's Sleep Habits Questionnaire (CSHQ): Psychometric Properties of a Survey Instrument for School-Aged Children. *Sleep* 23, no. 8 (2000): 1043–51.

    Goodlin-Jones, B. L., Sitnick, S. L., Tang, K., Liu, J., and Anders, T. F. "The Children's Sleep Habits Questionnaire in Toddlers and Preschool Children." *Journal of Developmental and Behavioral Pediatrics* 29, no. 2 (2008): 82–88.

- ***Pediatric Sleep Questionnaire.*** (Chervin et al., 2000). This is a parent-report measure of behaviors related to sleep-disordered breathing in children and adolescents ages 2 to 18 years of age.
  Chervin, R. D., Hedger, K., Dillon, J. E., Pituch, K. J. "Pediatric Sleep Questionnaire (PSQ): Validity and Reliability of Scales for Sleep-Disordered Breathing, Snoring, Sleepiness, and Behavioral Problems." *Sleep Medicine Reviews* 1, no. 1 (2000): 21–32.

- ***Sleep Disturbance Scale for Children.*** (Bruni et al., 1996). Parents of children ages 5 to 15 years of age are asked about medical and behavioral aspects of their children's sleep.
  Bruni, O., Ottaviano, S., Guidetti, V., Romoli, M., Innocenzi, M., Cortesi, F., and Giannotti, F. "The Sleep Disturbance Scale for Children (SDSC): Construction and Validation of an Instrument to Evaluate Sleep Disturbances in Childhood and Adolescence." *Journal of Sleep Research* 5, no. 4 (1996): 251–61.

- ***Sleep Habits Survey.*** (Wolfson et al., 2003). Children and adolescents ages 10 to 19 years of age are asked to report on their sleep difficulties.
  Wolfson, A. R., Carskadon, M. A., Acebo, C., Seifer, R., Fallone, G., Labyak, S. E., and Martin, J. L. "Evidence for the Validity of a Sleep Habits Survey for Adolescents." *Sleep* 26, no. 2 (2003): 213–16.

- ***Sleep Self Report.*** (Owens et al., 2000). This measure asks children ages 7 to 12 to report on their sleep habits and difficulties.
  Owens, J. A., Maxim, R., Nobile, C., McGuinn, M., and Msall, M. "Parental and Self-Report of Sleep in Children with Attention-Deficit/Hyperactivity Disorder." *Archives of Pediatric Adolescent Medicine* 154, no. 6 (2000): 549–55.

Appendix B
The BEARS Sleep Screening Tool

This brief questionnaire will help you determine if your child has sleep difficulties that should be addressed. After each set of questions, we have included references to relevant sections in this book.

B = bedtime problems
E = excessive daytime sleepiness
A = awakenings during the night
R = regularity and duration of sleep
S = snoring

	Toddler/ preschool (2–5 years)	**School-aged (6–12 years)**	**Adolescent (13–18 years)**
Bedtime problems	Does your child have any problems going to bed? Falling asleep?	Does your child have any problems at bedtime? (P)* Do you have any problems going to bed? (C)*	Do you have any problems falling asleep at bedtime? (C)
Why do these questions matter? (Chapter 2, 5) *What can you do? (Chapter 5, 6)*			
Excessive daytime sleepiness	Does your child seem overtired or sleep a lot during the day? Does she still take naps?	Does your child have difficulty working in the morning, seem sleepy during the day, or take naps? (P) Do you feel tired a lot? (C)	Do you feel sleepy a lot during the day? In school? While driving? (C)
Why do these questions matter? (Chapter 2, 5) *What can you do? (Chapter 5, 6, 7)*			

(Additional copies of this worksheet may be downloaded or printed from www.woodbinehouse.com/SolvingSleepProblems.asp)

Awakenings during the night	Does your child wake up a lot at night?	Does your child seem to wake up a lot at night? Any sleep walking or nightmares? (P) Do you wake up a lot at night? Have trouble getting back to sleep? (C)	Do you wake up a lot at night? Have trouble going back to sleep? (C)
Why do these questions matter? (Chapters 2, 5) *What can you do? (Chapters 5, 6, 7)*			
Regularity and duration of sleep	Does your child have a regular bedtime and wake time? What are they?	What time does your child go to bed and get up on school days? Weekends? Do you think he/she is getting enough sleep? (P)	What time do you usually go to bed on school nights? Weekends? How much sleep do you usually get? (C)
Why do these questions matter? (Chapter 2, 4) *What can you do? (Chapter 5, 6, 7)*			
Snoring/sleep disordered breathing	Does your child snore a lot or have difficulty breathing at night?	Does your child have loud or nightly snoring or any breathing difficulties at night? (P)	Does your teenager snore loudly or nightly? (P)
Why do these questions matter? (Chapter 2, 5) *What can you do? (Chapter 5)*			

*P = question for parents; C = question for child

From Owens, J. A., and Alzell, V. "Use of the 'BEARS' Sleep Screening Tool in a Pediatric Residents' Continuity Clinic: A Pilot Study." *Sleep Medicine* 6, no. 1 (2005): 63–69.

Appendix C

Children's Sleep Habits Questionnaire

SECTION B: SURVEY ITEMS						
Bedtime Information			**Time (e.g., 12:00)**			
1.	During the week what time does your child usually go to sleep?		x : xx			☐am ☐pm
2.	During the week what time does your child usually wake up?		x : xx			☐am ☐pm
3.	On the weekend what time does your child usually go to sleep?		x : xx			☐am ☐pm
4.	On the weekend what time does your child usually wake up?		x : xx			☐am ☐pm

Please answer both questions for each item: a. How often? and b. Is it a problem?	**a. How often?** rarely (0–1)	sometimes (2–4)	usually (5–7)	**b. Is it a problem?** NO	YES
5. Child goes to bed at the same time at night	☐	☐	☐	☐	☐
6. Child falls asleep within 20 minutes after going to bed	☐	☐	☐	☐	☐
7. Child falls asleep alone in own bed	☐	☐	☐	☐	☐
8. Child falls asleep in parent's or sibling's bed	☐	☐	☐	☐	☐
9. Child needs parent in the room to fall asleep	☐	☐	☐	☐	☐
10. Child struggles at bedtime (cries, refuses to stay in bed, etc.)	☐	☐	☐	☐	☐
11. Child is afraid of sleeping in the dark	☐	☐	☐	☐	☐
12. Child is afraid of sleeping alone	☐	☐	☐	☐	☐

(Additional copies of this worksheet may be downloaded or printed from www.woodbinehouse.com/SolvingSleepProblems.asp)

Sleep Behavior

13. Child's usual amount of sleep each day (combining night time sleep and naps):

____ Hours ___ Minutes

Please answer both questions for each item: a. How often? and b. Is it a problem?	**a. How often?**			**b. Is it a problem?**	
	rarely (0–1)	**sometimes (2–4)**	**usually (5–7)**	**NO**	**YES**
14. Child sleeps too little	☐	☐	☐	☐	☐
15. Child sleeps the right amount	☐	☐	☐	☐	☐
16. Child sleeps about the same amount each day	☐	☐	☐	☐	☐
17. Child wets the bed at night	☐	☐	☐	☐	☐
18. Child talks during sleep	☐	☐	☐	☐	☐
19. Child is restless and moves a lot during sleep	☐	☐	☐	☐	☐
20. Child sleepwalks during the night	☐	☐	☐	☐	☐
21. Child moves to someone else's bed during the night (parent, brother, sister, etc.)	☐	☐	☐	☐	☐
22. Child grinds teeth during sleep (dentist may have told you this)	☐	☐	☐	☐	☐
23. Child snores loudly	☐	☐	☐	☐	☐
24. Child seems to stop breathing during sleep	☐	☐	☐	☐	☐
25. Child snorts and/or gasps during sleep	☐	☐	☐	☐	☐
26. Child has trouble sleeping away from home (visiting relatives, vacation, etc.)	☐	☐	☐	☐	☐
27. Child awakens during the night screaming, sweating, and inconsolable	☐	☐	☐	☐	☐
28. Child awakens alarmed by a frightening dream	☐	☐	☐	☐	☐

Waking During the Night *Please answer both questions for each item:* *a. How often? and b. Is it a problem?*	**a. How often?** **rarely (0–1)**	**sometimes (2–4)**	**usually (5–7)**	**b. Is it a problem?** **NO**	**YES**
29. Child awakes once during the night	☐	☐	☐	☐	☐
30. Child awakes more than once during the night	☐	☐	☐	☐	☐
31. Write the number of minutes a night waking usually lasts: *(If they do not wake during the night, please record 0 min.)*	0 minutes				

Morning Waking/Daytime Sleepiness *Please answer both questions for each item:* *a. How often? and b. Is it a problem?*	**a. How often?** **rarely (0–1)**	**sometimes (2–4)**	**usually (5–7)**	**b. Is it a problem?** **NO**	**YES**
32. Child wakes up by him/herself	☐	☐	☐	☐	☐
33. Child wakes up in negative mood	☐	☐	☐	☐	☐
34. Adults or siblings wake up child	☐	☐	☐	☐	☐
35. Child has difficulty getting out of bed in the morning	☐	☐	☐	☐	☐
36. Child takes a long time to become alert in the morning	☐	☐	☐	☐	☐
37. Child seems tired	☐	☐	☐	☐	☐

Child has appeared very sleepy / fallen asleep during the following:	**not sleepy**	**very sleepy**	**falls asleep**	**not applicable**
38. …watching TV	☐	☐	☐	☐
39. …riding in car	☐	☐	☐	☐

The questionnaire included here is a shortened version of the CSHQ, modified from the survey originally published in the following:

Owens, J. A., Spirito, A., McGuinn, M., and Nobile, C. "Sleep Habits and Sleep Disturbance in Elementary School-Aged Children." *Journal of Developmental and Behavioral Pediatrics* 21, no. 1 (2000), 27–36.

To help you decide if your child has difficulties with sleep and to guide you in making changes in her sleep habits, you can go through the Child Sleep Habits Questionnaire (CSHQ) question by question below. We have included references to related sections in this book after each question so that you can learn more about why this question is important and what steps you can take to make things better.

Bedtime Information

1. During the week what time does your child usually go to sleep?
   Why does this matter? (Chapter 2, 4)
   What can you do about it? (Chapter 5, 6, 7)

2. During the week what time does your child usually wake up?
   Why does this matter? (Chapter 2, 4)
   What can you do about it? (Chapter 5, 6, 7)

3. On the weekend what time does your child usually go to sleep?
   Why does this matter? (Chapter 2, 4)
   What can you do about it? (Chapter 5, 6, 7)

4. On the weekend what time does your child usually wake up?
   Why does this matter? (Chapter 2, 4, 5)
   What can you do about it? (Chapter 5, 6, 7)

5. Child goes to bed at the same time at night
   Why does this matter? (Chapter 4)
   What can you do about it? Chapter 6, 7)

6. Child falls asleep within 20 minutes after going to bed
   Why does this matter? (Chapter 2, 4, 5)
   What can you do about it? (Chapter 5, 6, 7)

7. Child falls asleep alone in own bed
   Why does this matter? (Chapter 4)
   What can you do about it? (Chapter 6, 7)

8. Child falls asleep in parent's or sibling's bed
   Why does this matter? (Chapter 4)
   What can you do about it? (Chapter 6, 7)

9. Child needs parent in the room to fall asleep
   Why does this matter? (Chapter 4)
   What can you do about it? (Chapter 6, 7)

10. Child struggles at bedtime (cries, refuses to stay in bed, etc.)
    Why does this matter? (Chapter 4)
    What can you do about it? (Chapter 6, 7)

11. Child is afraid of sleeping in the dark
    Why does this matter? (Chapter 4)
    What can you do about it? (Chapter 6, 7)

12. Child is afraid of sleeping alone
    Why does this matter? (Chapter 4)
    What can you do about it? (Chapter 6, 7)

13. What is the child's usual amount of sleep?
    Why does this matter? (Chapter 1)
    What can you do about it? (Chapter 6, 7)

Sleep Behavior

14. Child sleeps too little
    Why does this matter? (Chapter 1, 2, 5)
    What can you do about it? (Chapter 5, 6, 7)

15. Child sleeps the right amount
    Why does this matter? (Chapter 1, 2)
    What can you do about it? (Chapter 5, 6, 7)

16. Child sleeps about the same amount each day
    Why does this matter? (Chapter 2)
    What can you do about it? (Chapter 5, 6, 7)

17. Child wets the bed at night
    Why does this matter? (Chapter 7)
    What can you do about it? (Chapter 7)

18. Child talks during sleep
    Why does this matter? (Chapter 5)
    What can you do about it? (Chapter 5, 7)

19. Child is restless and moves a lot during sleep
    Why does this matter? (Chapter 5)
    What can you do about it? (Chapter 5, 6)

20. Child sleepwalks during the night
    Why does this matter? (Chapter 5)
    What can you do about it? (Chapter 5, 7)

21. Child moves to someone else's bed during the night (a parent, brother, sister, or other family member)
    Why does this matter? (Chapter 4, 5)
    What can you do about it? (Chapter 6, 7)

22. Child grinds teeth during sleep (dentist may have told you this)
    Why does this matter? (Chapter 5)
    What can you do about it? (Chapter 5)

23. Child snores loudly
    Why does this matter? (Chapter 5)
    What can you do about it? (Chapter 5)

24. Child seems to stop breathing during sleep
    Why does this matter? (Chapter 5)
    What can you do about it? (Chapter 5)

25. Child snorts and/or gasps during sleep
    Why does this matter? (Chapter 5)
    What can you do about it? (Chapter 5)

26. Child has trouble sleeping away from home (visiting relatives, vacation, etc.)
    Why does this matter? (Chapter 9)
    What can you do about it? (Chapter 9)

27. Child awakens during the night screaming, sweating, and inconsolable
    Why does this matter? (Chapter 5)
    What can you do about it? (Chapter 5)

28. Child awakens alarmed by a frightening dream
    Why does this matter? (Chapter 7)
    What can you do about it? (Chapter 7)

Waking During the Night

29. Child awakes once during the night
    Why does this matter? (Chapter 4, 5)
    What can you do about it? (Chapter 5, 6, 7)

30. Child awakes more than once during the night
    Why does this matter? (Chapter 4, 5)
    What can you do about it? (Chapter 5, 6, 7)

31. Write the number of minutes a night waking usually lasts:
    Why does this matter? (Chapter 4, 5)
    What can you do about it? (Chapter 5, 6, 7)

Morning Waking/Daytime Sleepiness

32. Child wakes up by him- or herself
    Why does this matter? (Chapter 4, 5)
    What can you do about it? (Chapter 5, 6, 7)

33. Child wakes up in negative mood
    Why does this matter? (Chapter 4, 5)
    What can you do about it? (Chapter 5, 6, 7)

34. Adults or siblings wake up child
    Why does this matter? (Chapter 4, 5)
    What can you do about it? (Chapter 5, 6, 7)

35. Child has difficulty getting out of bed in the morning
    Why does this matter? (Chapter 4, 5)
    What can you do about it? (Chapter 5, 6, 7)

36. Child takes a long time to become alert in the morning
    Why does this matter? (Chapter 4, 5)
    What can you do about it? (Chapter 5, 6, 7)

37. Child seems tired
    Why does this matter? (Chapter 4, 5)
    What can you do about it? (Chapter 5, 6, 7)

38. Child has appeared very sleepy/fallen asleep during the following:
    ...watching TV
    ...riding in car
    Why does this matter? (Chapter 4, 5)
    What can you do about it? (Chapter 4, 5, 6, 7)

Appendix D

Family Inventory of Sleep Habits (FISH)

Date: ____________________

Name of Child: ____________________

Relationship to Child: ____________________

DIRECTIONS: For each item below, please indicate how often it was true within the last month. Please answer each question below. If multiple choices are available, please select one answer.

	Never 1	Occasionally 2	Sometimes 3	Usually 4	Always 5
1. My child gets exercise during the day.	☐	☐	☐	☐	☐
2. My child naps more than one hour during the day.	☐	☐	☐	☐	☐
3. My child's bedroom is used as a "time-out" area for discipline during the day.	☐	☐	☐	☐	☐
4. My child's bedroom is used as a play area during the day.	☐	☐	☐	☐	☐
5. My child wakes up at about the same time each morning.	☐	☐	☐	☐	☐
6. In the hour before bedtime, my child engages in relaxing activities.	☐	☐	☐	☐	☐
7. My child has drinks or foods with caffeine after 5 p.m. (e.g., chocolate, soda).	☐	☐	☐	☐	☐
8. In the hour before bedtime, my child engages in exciting or stimulating activities (e.g., rough play, video games, sports).	☐	☐	☐	☐	☐
9. My child sleeps better when wearing pajamas/sleepwear made from certain fabric(s).	☐	☐	☐	☐	☐

(Additional copies of this worksheet may be downloaded or printed from www.woodbinehouse.com/SolvingSleepProblems.asp)

	Never 1	Occasionally 2	Sometimes 3	Usually 4	Always 5
10. My child sleeps better with certain sheets or blankets on his/her bed.	☐	☐	☐	☐	☐
11. My child sleeps better when his/her room is a certain temperature at night (either warm or cool).	☐	☐	☐	☐	☐
12. My child's room is dark or dimly lit at bedtime.	☐	☐	☐	☐	☐
13. My child's room is quiet at bedtime.	☐	☐	☐	☐	☐
14. My child goes to bed at the same time each night.	☐	☐	☐	☐	☐
15. My child follows a regular bedtime routine that lasts 15-30 minutes.	☐	☐	☐	☐	☐
16. My child has a favorite comfort object that he/she sleeps with.	☐	☐	☐	☐	☐
17. I stay in my child's room until he/she falls asleep.	☐	☐	☐	☐	☐
18. After my child is tucked in, I check on him/her before he/she falls asleep.	☐	☐	☐	☐	☐
19. My child watches TV, videos, or DVDs to help him/her fall asleep.	☐	☐	☐	☐	☐
20. My child listens to music to help him/her fall asleep.	☐	☐	☐	☐	☐
21. If my child wakes up during the night, I keep our interactions brief. ➢ ***If your child does not wake up during the night, check here:*** ☐ ***N/A***	☐	☐	☐	☐	☐
22. If my child gets out of bed during the night, I return my child to his/her bed. ➢ ***If your child does not get out of bed during the night, check here:*** ☐ ***N/A***	☐	☐	☐	☐	☐

To help you understand and follow-up on your answers to the Family Inventory of Sleep Habits (FISH), you may refer to the pages in this book that are listed after each question.

1. My child gets exercise during the day.
   Why does this matter? (page 29)
   What can you do about it? (page 52)

2. My child naps more than one hour during the day.
   Why does this matter? (page 32)
   What can you do about it? (pages 54, 98)

3. My child's bedroom is used as a "time-out" area for discipline during the day.
   Why does this matter? (pages 30-32)
   What can you do about it? (pages 55-56)

4. My child's bedroom is used as a play area during the day.
   Why does this matter? (page 30)
   What can you do about it? (pages 55-56)

5. My child wakes up at about the same time each morning.
   Why does this matter? (pages 21-22)
   What can you do about it? (page 72)

6. In the hour before bedtime, my child engages in relaxing activities.
   Why does this matter? (pages 32-33)
   What can you do about it? (pages 57-58, 64, 71, 81)

7. My child has drinks or foods with caffeine after 5 p.m. (e.g., chocolate, soda).
   Why does this matter? (page 30)
   What can you do about it? (pages 53-54)

8. In the hour before bedtime, my child engages in exciting or stimulating activities (e.g., rough play, video games, sports).
   Why does this matter? (pages 32-33)
   What can you do about it? (pages 57, 64)

9. My child sleeps better when wearing pajamas/sleepwear made from certain fabric(s).
   Why does this matter? (page 35)
   What can you do about it? (pages 76-77)

10. My child sleeps better with certain sheets or blankets on his/her bed.
   Why does this matter? (page 35)
   What can you do about it? (pages 76-77)

11. My child sleeps better when his/her room is a certain temperature at night (either warm or cool).
   Why does this matter? (page 35)
   What can you do about it? (page 76)

12. My child's room is dark or dimly lit at bedtime.
   Why does this matter? (pages 29, 33, 36)
   What can you do about it? (pages 59-60, 78, 97, 103)

13. My child's room is quiet at bedtime.
   Why does this matter? (page 36)
   What can you do about it? (pages 77-78)

14. My child goes to bed at the same time each night.
   Why does this matter? (pages 21, 72)
   What can you do about it? (pages 72, 73)

15. My child follows a regular bedtime routine that lasts 15–30 minutes.
   Why does this matter? (pages 16, 34, 60)
   What can you do about it? (pages 60-69)

16. My child has a favorite comfort object that he/she sleeps with.
   Why does this matter? (pages 26, 27)
   What can you do about it? (page 86)

17. I stay in my child's room until he/she falls asleep.
   Why does this matter? (page 26)
   What can you do about it? (pages 86-87)

18. After my child is tucked in, I check on him/her before he/she falls asleep.
   Why does this matter? (page 26)
   What can you do about it? (pages 85, 99)

19. My child watches TV, videos, or DVDs to help him/her fall asleep.
    Why does this matter? (pages 25, 27, 83-84)
    What can you do about it? (pages 59, 78, 96)

20. My child listens to music to help him/her fall asleep.
    Why does this matter? (page 27)
    What can you do about it? (pages 77, 87)

21. If my child wakes up during the night, I keep our interactions brief.
    Why does this matter? (page 28)
    What can you do about it? (pages 85, 90, 92)

22. If my child gets out of bed during the night, I return my child to his/her bed.
    Why does this matter? (pages 27, 28)
    What can you do about it? (pages 87, 89, 91, 92)

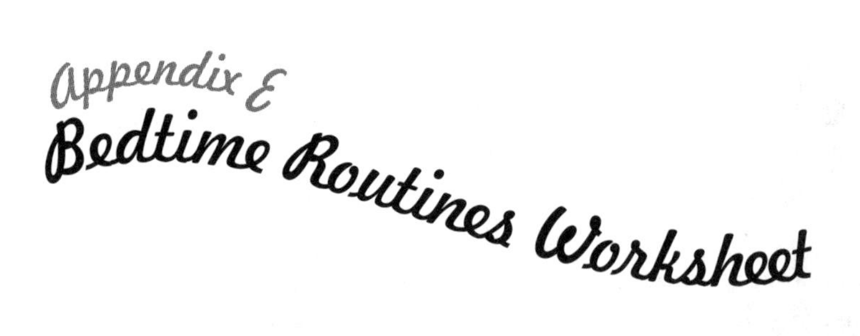

Activities	Occurs	Is the activity easy (E) or hard (H)?	Is the activity stimulating (S) or relaxing (R)?	Rank in order of preference (1, 2, 3)
Taking a bath				
Washing hair				
Changing into pajamas				
Getting a drink				
Brushing teeth				
Using the bathroom				
Singing quiet songs				
Reading				
Other:				

Bedtime Schedule

Using the information from the Bedtime Routines Worksheet, plan a bedtime schedule for your child.

Order	Activity	Is the activity easy (E) or hard (H)?	Is the activity stimulating (S) or relaxing (R)?

(Additional copies of this worksheet may be downloaded or printed from www.woodbinehouse.com/SolvingSleepProblems.asp)

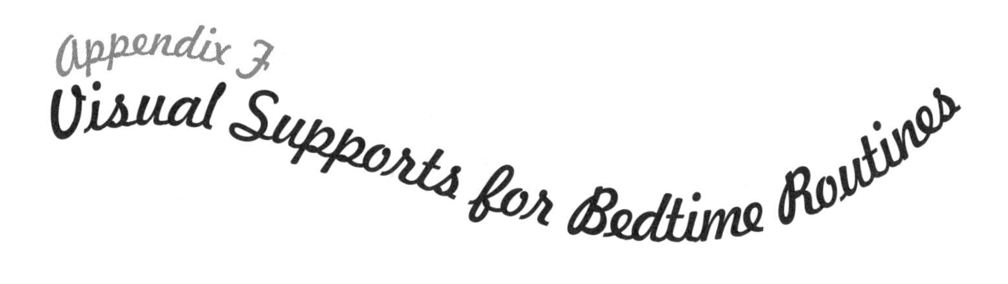

Appendix 7
Visual Supports for Bedtime Routines

Brush
Brush teeth
Choices
Draw
Eat a snack
Get a drink
Go to bed
Go to sleep
Go to the bathroom

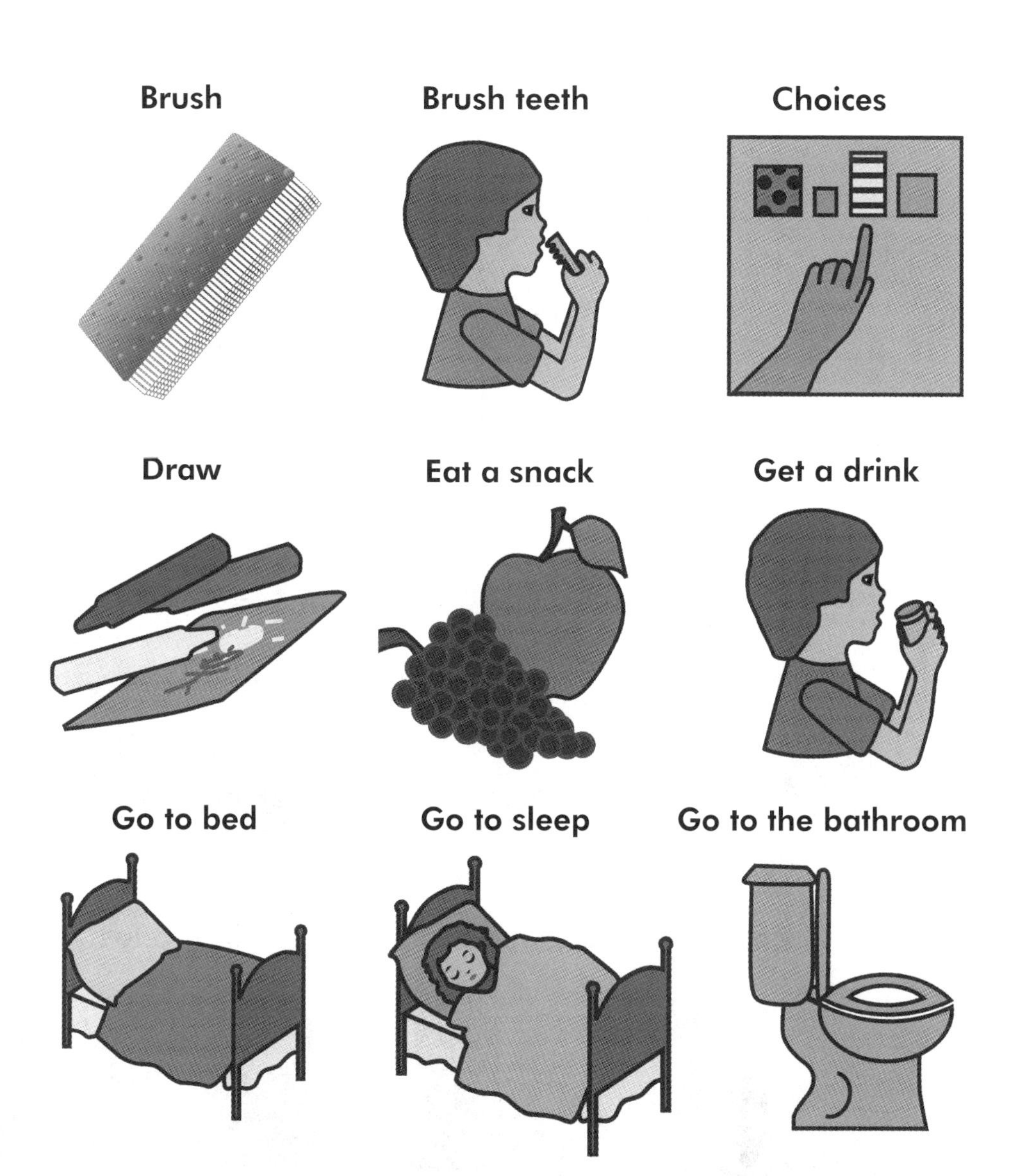

(Additional copies of this worksheet may be downloaded or printed from www.woodbinehouse.com/SolvingSleepProblems.asp)

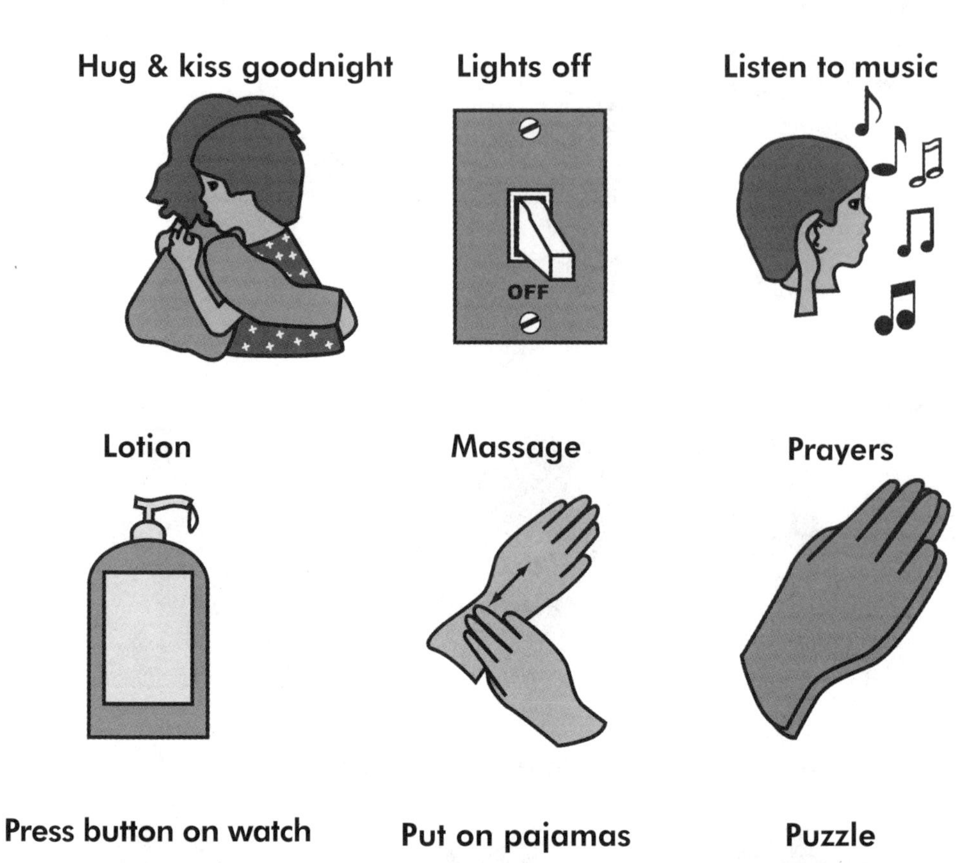

Press button on watch

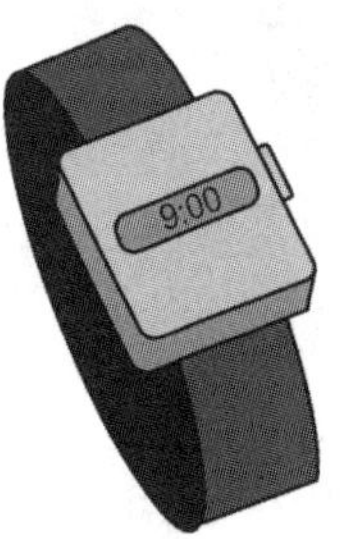

Put on pajamas

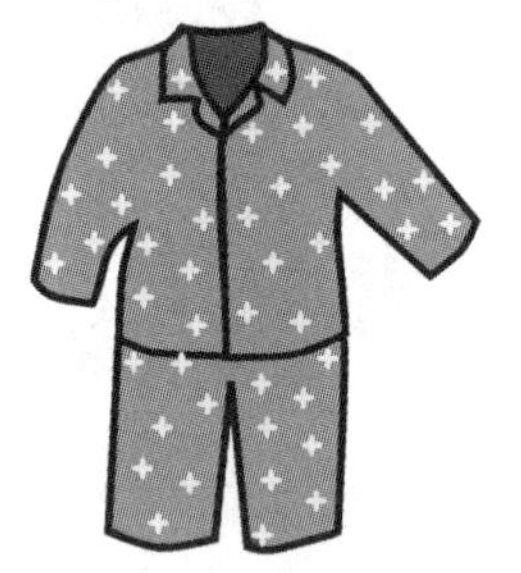

Puzzle

Read a book

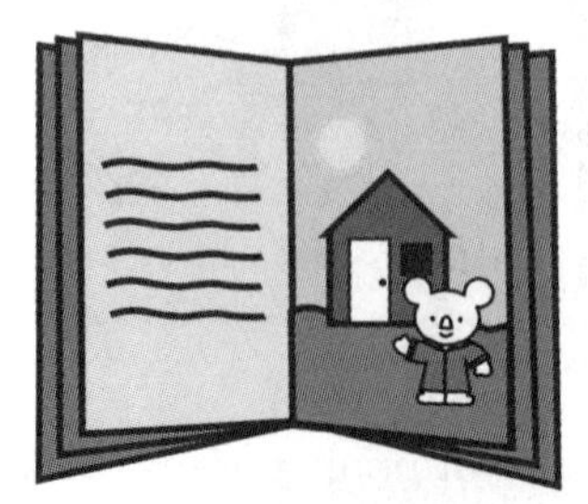

Rocking chair

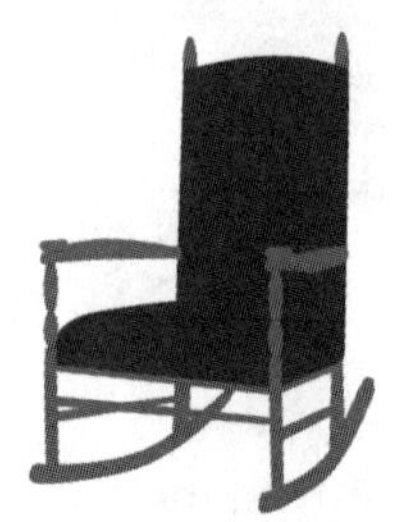

Sing songs

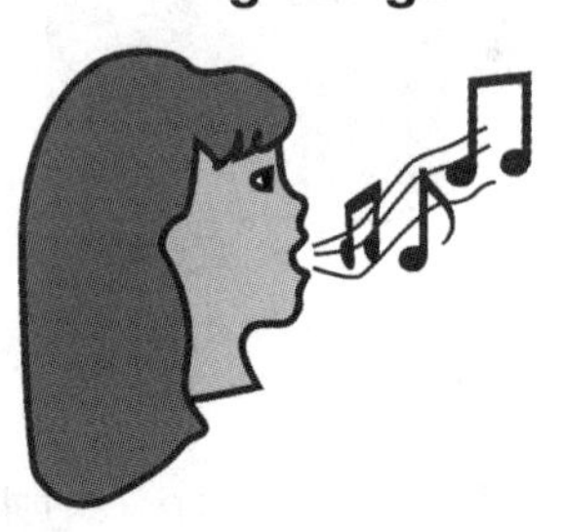

Take a bath

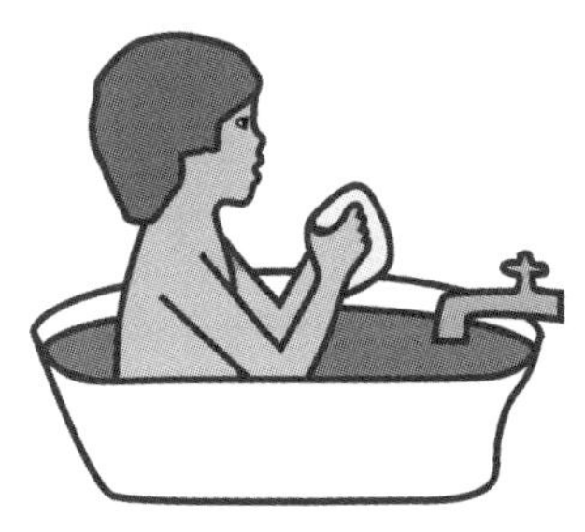

Take a shower

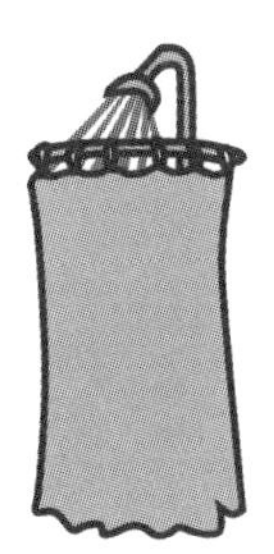

Take medicine

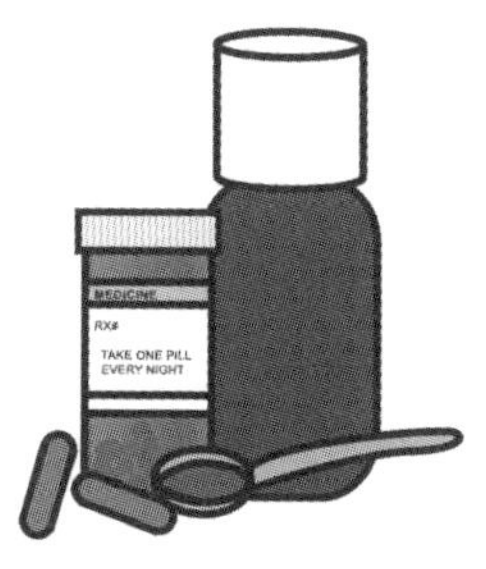

Wash face & hands

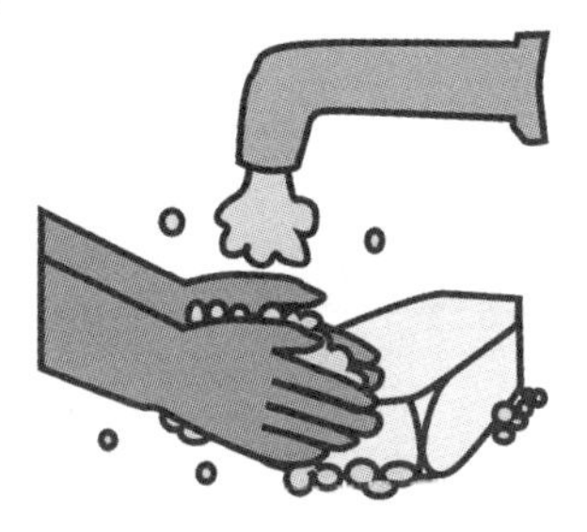

Wash hair

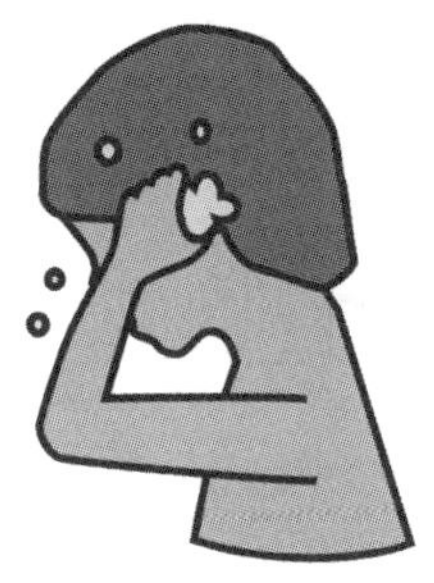

Weighted blanket

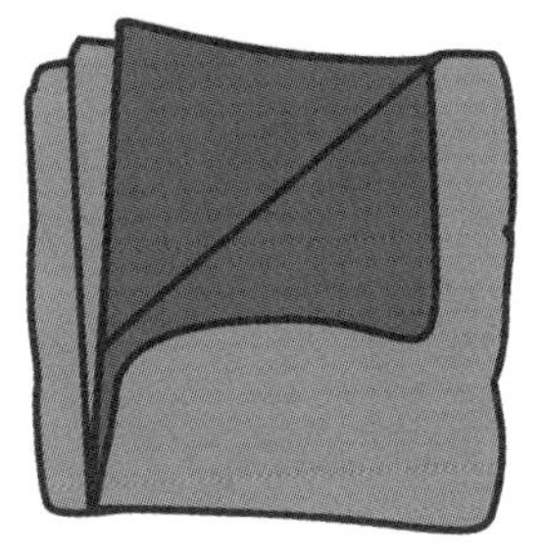

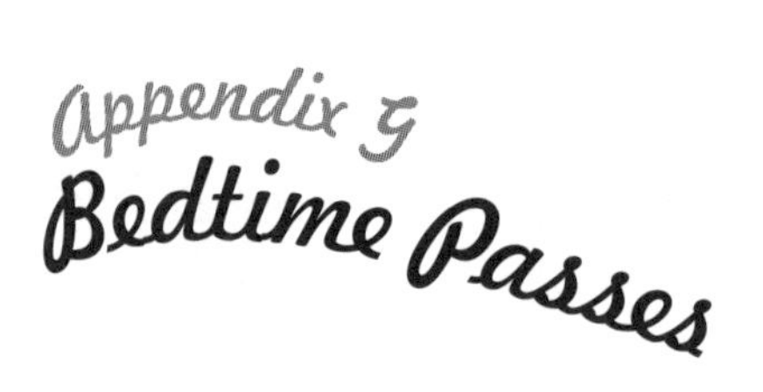

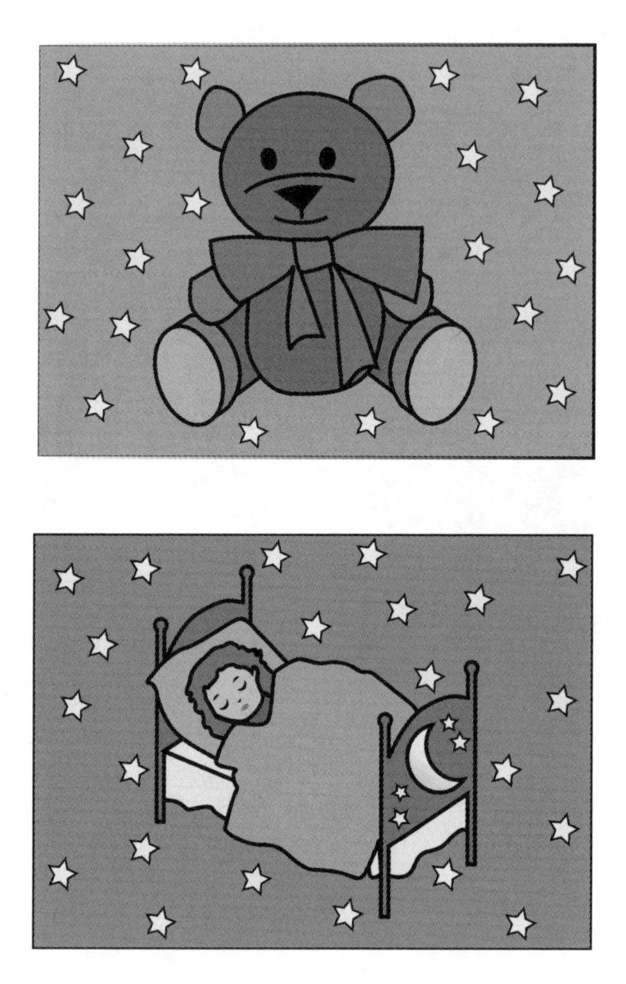

(Additional copies of this worksheet may be downloaded or printed from www.woodbinehouse.com/SolvingSleepProblems.asp)

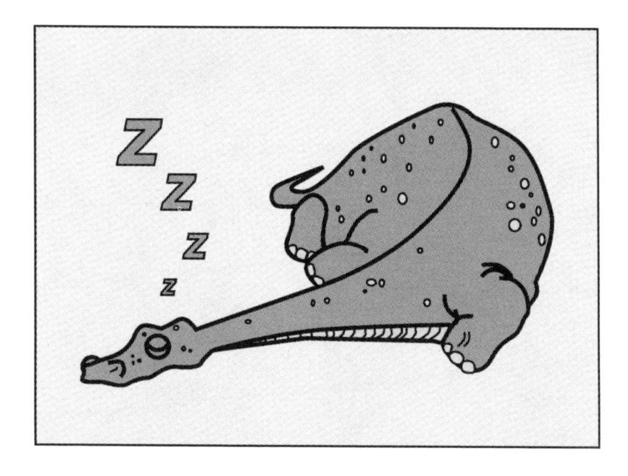

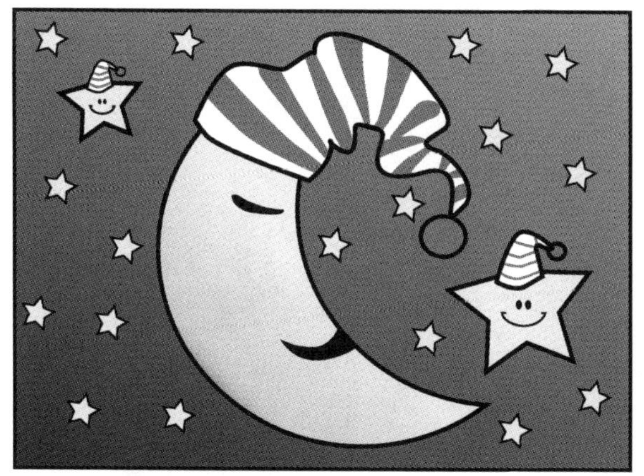

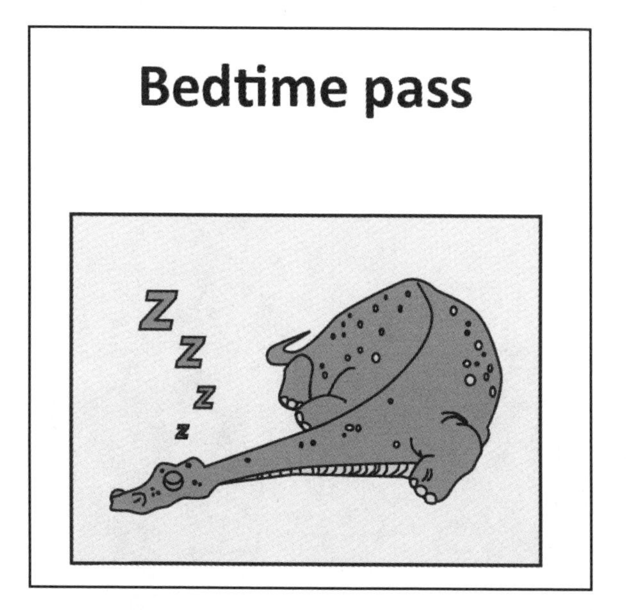
Bedtime pass

Appendix H Sleep Record

	Date:	Date:	Date:	Date:	Date:	Date:	Date:
Daytime Habits	Minutes spent in: Exercise ___	Minutes spent in: Exercise ___	Minutes spent in: Exercise:___	Minutes spent in: Exercise:___	Minutes spent in: Exercise:___	Minutes spent in: Exercise ___	Minutes spent in: Exercise ___
	Naps ______	Naps ______	Naps ______	Naps ______	Naps ______	Naps ______	Naps ______
Caffeine	Amount (mg)_____	Amount (mg)_____	Amount (mg)_____	Amount (mg)_____	Amount (mg)_____	Amount (mg)_____	Amount (mg)_____
Morning Light?	___Yes ___No	___Yes ___No	___Yes ___No	___Yes ___No	___Yes ___No	___Yes ___No	___Yes ___No
Evening Activities (stop time)	Dinner ___pm Homework ___ pm TV/videos ___pm Video games __pm Exercise ___pm Other ___pm	Dinner ___pm Homework ___ pm TV/videos ___pm Video games __pm Exercise ___pm Other ___pm	Dinner ___pm Homework ___ pm TV/videos ___pm Video games __pm Exercise ___pm Other ___pm	Dinner ___pm Homework ___ pm TV/videos ___pm Video games __pm Exercise ___pm Other ___pm	Dinner ___pm Homework ___ pm TV/videos ___pm Video games __pm Exercise ___pm Other ___pm	Dinner ___pm Homework ___ pm TV/videos ___pm Videogames __pm Exercise ___pm Other ___pm	Dinner ___pm Homework ___ pm TV/videos ___pm Video games __pm Exercise ___pm Other ___pm
Sleep Setting	Any Problems? Location	Problems with: Location	Problems with: Location	Problems with: Location	Problems with: Location	Problems with: Location	Problems with: Location

	Temperature Texture Scents Sounds Light Objects	Temperature Texture Scents Sounds Light Objects	Temperature Texture Scents Sounds Light Objects	Temperature Texture Scents Sounds Light Objects	Temperature Texture Scents Sounds Light Objects	Temperature Texture Scents Sounds Light Objects	Temperature Texture Scents Sounds Light Objects
Bedtime Routine	Start time ___pm Activities include: 1. 2. 3. 4. 5. 6. 7.	Start time ___pm Activities include: 1. 2. 3. 4. 5. 6. 7.	Start time ___pm Activities include: 1. 2. 3. 4. 5. 6. 7.	Start time ___pm Activities include: 1. 2. 3. 4. 5. 6. 7.	Start time ___pm Activities include: 1. 2. 3. 4. 5. 6. 7.	Start time ___pm Activities include: 1. 2. 3. 4. 5. 6. 7.	Start time ___pm Activities include: 1. 2. 3. 4. 5. 6. 7.

Visual supports?	Yes No	Yes No	Yes No	Yes No	Yes No	Yes No	Yes No
Bedtime	____pm	____pm	____pm	____pm	____pm	____pm	____pm
How long to fall asleep?							
Sleep Resistance Strategies (circle what you have tried)	Crying it out Checking in Rocking chair Morning presents Delay bedtime	Crying it out Checking in Rocking chair Morning presents Delay bedtime	Crying it out Checking in Rocking chair Morning presents Delay bedtime	Crying it out Checking in Rocking chair Morning presents Delay bedtime	Crying it out Checking in Rocking chair Morning presents Delay bedtime	Crying it out Checking in Rocking chair Morning presents Delay bedtime	Crying it out Checking in Rocking chair Morning presents Delay bedtime
Night Wakings	How many___	How many___	How many___	How many___	How many___	How many___	How many___
	How long___	How long___	How long___	How long___	How long___	How long___	How long___
	Child leave bed? Yes__ No__	Child leave bed? Yes__ No__	Child leave bed? Yes__ No__	Child leave bed? Yes__ No__	Child leave bed? Yes__ No__	Child leave bed? Yes__ No__	Child leave bed? Yes__ No__
Your Response?							
Wake Time	___am	___am	___am	___am	___am	___am	___am

Index

About the Authors

Jerry Katz, a licensed psychologist, has worked with children with ASD for over 25 years. She is the co-founder of an ASD sleep clinic at the Child Development Unit, Children's Hospital Colorado, Department of Pediatrics Section of Neurodevelopmental and Behavioral Pediatrics, University of Colorado School of Medicine. Dr. Katz is also on the faculty at JFK Partners, University of Colorado School of Medicine, Colorado's University Center of Excellence in Developmental Disabilities (UCEDD) and Leadership Education in Neurodevelopmental Disabilities (LEND) Program. Her research focuses on sleep difficulties in children with ASD.

Beth Malow, Burry Chair in Cognitive Childhood Development, and Professor of Neurology and Pediatrics at Vanderbilt University, is a sleep neurologist with expertise in ASD. The focus of Dr. Malow's research is on treatments of sleep disorders in ASD, with an emphasis toward behavioral approaches. She is also the parent of two children with ASD, and brings this valuable perspective to her work.